Integrating the Participants' Perspective in the Study of Language and Communication Disorders

"Involvement of participants in research and in person-centered care delivery poses challenges—at experiential, ontological and epistemological levels. In her integrationist endeavor, Klemmensen shifts from a deficit ideology underpinning language/communication disorder studies by pointing to the 'competence gap' of the researcher-analysts and the attendant disciplines in their sense-making practices. The book's merits include breadth of coverage, deeply engaging argumentation and the overall attempt at integrating not only different conceptual/ analytical frameworks but also the diverse readership."

—Srikant Sarangi, *Professor in Humanities and Medicine, Director, Danish Institute of Humanities and Medicine, Aalborg University, Denmark*

"In this profoundly challenging work Klemmensen poses fundamental questions about the ability of our models of language and communication to do justice to the study of language disorders. Underlying the discussion are the most basic questions that confront the study of human interaction, namely those of description and explanation within competing theoretical frameworks, the nature of norms and regularities, the grounds of professional expertise and outsider insight, the ethics of reduction in analysis, and our ability to grasp the lived experience and communicational competences of the participants themselves."

—Christopher Hutton, *Chair Professor, School of English, The University of Hong Kong, China*

Charlotte Marie Bisgaard Klemmensen

Integrating the Participants' Perspective in the Study of Language and Communication Disorders

Towards a New Analytical Approach

palgrave
macmillan

Charlotte Marie Bisgaard Klemmensen
Department of Communication
  and Psychology
Aalborg University
Aalborg, Denmark

ISBN 978-3-319-78633-9   ISBN 978-3-319-78634-6 (eBook)
https://doi.org/10.1007/978-3-319-78634-6

Library of Congress Control Number: 2018937865

Cover illustration: © John Rawsterne/patternhead.com

Printed on acid-free paper

This Palgrave Pivot imprint is published by the registered company Springer
International Publishing AG part of Springer Nature
The registered company address is: Gewerbestrasse 11, 6330 Cham, Switzerland

To my mother, who had two strokes of cerebral apoplexy, and my father

PREFACE

This preface introduces the organization of the book. It is built around an interdisciplinary analytical framework which enhances the understanding of individuals with communication deficiencies, such as linguistic impairments and aphasia following acquired brain injury. It is structured as a short monograph and offers an overall discussion of contemporary widely discussed approaches to the study of the practices of everyday life. The scope of the book extends far beyond the study of language and communication disorders. There are several groups in the intended audience: students, practicing health professionals, and interested lay-persons. The intended academic audience consists of scholars and graduate students investigating the atypical communication in the fields of applied linguistics, interaction studies, social psychology using the approaches of ethnomethodology, conversation analysis, social constructionism, constructivism, practice studies, practice theory, and discourse studies. Additionally, peer researchers and students interested in probing an applied integrational linguistic perspective are targeted. New entanglements of theoretical perspectives are presented mainly to scholars, and students will find a moment to explore the development of a new analytical perspective in the making.

The content of the book is relevant to the educational training of health and social care professionals. It is also relevant for practitioners already in the field and for professionals planning supervision. Finally, it may be interesting to non-professionals, for instance family members related to individuals with conditions of language and communication disorders. In particular, it may be of interest to the topic's narrators: it might add or develop an already present self-awareness of the disorder-perspective for individuals living with language and communication disorders.

Chapters 2–4 have been written for non-expert readers: they offer accessible accounts of current research and approaches to the study of meaning-making in practice. They introduce basic ideas of communication and practice turns. These introductory chapters survey the current state of the art. Chapters 5 and 6 introduce and probe a new analytical perspective: they merge a practice theoretical approach and an applied integrational linguistic perspective. Chapter 6 is where data are analyzed, and Chapter 7 concludes the overall idea of the new participants' perspective.

Aalborg, Denmark   Charlotte Marie Bisgaard Klemmensen

ACKNOWLEDGEMENTS

My thanks to Professor Pirkko Raudaskoski and Professor Srikant Sarangi at Aalborg University, and to Associate Professor Søren Beck Nielsen at University of Copenhagen for their expert guidance and help. Furthermore, I would like to thank Dr. Carrie Peterson, and my husband and children for their patience and tolerance.

CONTENTS

Contents

ABBREVIATIONS

ABI   Acquired brain injury
AR   Agential realism
CA   Conversation analysis
DP   Discursive psychology
EMCA   Ethnomethodology and conversation analysis program
ICF   International classification of functioning, disability and health
IL   Integrational linguistics
LCD   Language and communication disorder
NA   Nexus analysis
PT   Practice theory
QOL   Quality of life

LIST OF FIGURES

List of Figures

CHAPTER 1

Introduction

Abstract The chapter introduces the aim and topic of this book. Instances of recurring aphasia and acquired brain injury are discussed in an empirical observation study through a theoretical lens that combines integrational linguistics, ethnomethodology and conversation analysis, and practice theory. The integrational linguistic concept of integrational proficiency is foregrounded throughout this book by Harris (Integrationist notes and papers 2006–2008, Bright Pen, Gamlingay, 2009, p. 71). This study adds a person-centered perspective to existing ethnographic approaches. Thus, person-centeredness in an interaction analysis is discussed and applied in a way which invites scholars, professionals, and impaired individuals and their peers to refocus their perception of aphasia and acquired brain injury.

Keywords Interdisciplinarity · Analytical person-centeredness · Atypical communication · Integrationism · Practice studies · Revisit language disorders

This book proposes and discusses a novel analytical approach which contributes to the establishment of a new discourse in the study of communicational difficulties, traditionally known as the study of language disorders. The approach draws on the radical development into inquiry on language formulated by the late Oxford professor emeritus Roy

© The Author(s) 2018
C. M. B. Klemmensen, *Integrating the Participants' Perspective in the Study of Language and Communication Disorders*,
https://doi.org/10.1007/978-3-319-78634-6_1

Harris, who termed his approach integrationism (Harris 1996, 1998). In his book *The Language Myth* (1981), Harris initiated his program of demythologizing traditional Western assumptions about language and communication. In its pure form, Harris and fellow integrationists claim that integrationism has far-reaching implications for social, political, legal, philosophical, and psychological issues (www.integrationists. com). At best, over the past 40 years, integrationism has proved capable of defending the orthodox legacy of its own demythologizing practice. Consequently, not much interchange with the rest of the scientific community has taken place. This book aims to open this abandoned dialogue. The suggested new analytical approach frames an interdisciplinary perspective which combines basic assumptions of integrational linguistics (IL) with descriptive elements from the ethnomethodology and conversation analysis program (EMCA). These are joined in a framework on the grounds of the research agenda of practice theory (PT). As a result, an integrational practice perspective is conceptualized. This innovative approach allows new analytical insights to be gained. This book offers a fresh theoretical and methodological resource for further investigation of the social, relational, and communicational sides of linguistic impairment and aphasia following acquired brain injury (ABI).

This book's integrational stance contributes to the study of language and communication and adds an ontological fine-tuning to traditional interaction studies in aphasia. In an integrational practice perspective, social, relational, and communicational issues are considered to be present all the time, integrating a person's contextualization of real-life communication situations, including whenever impairment or ABI may emerge. Thus, this approach favors a new person-centeredness in interaction. As a consequence, the analysis focuses on the impaired individual's contextualization rather than on the social scene in isolation, which is richly covered by EMCA-approaches to interaction in ABI and aphasia.

The advances of this book lie in framing the new integrational practice perspective as an interdisciplinary perspective and in suggesting an implementation of it in the sub-areas of applied integrationism and health communication. Furthermore, it informs developers of quality of life (QOL) assessments with empirical insights into living with ABI and aphasia. Finally, it is a step towards offering a formative evaluation tool in health and social care. This book's idea of a new participant perspective distinctly affords an empirically based understanding of the individual, experiential side of ABI and aphasia.

Data are analyzed by switching lenses and by zooming in and out (Nicolini 2009). *Zooming in*, recorded moments of individuals in action in situated practices, is approached with analyses of the interaction. *Zooming out*, the discursive trajectories circulating the actual sites of engagements, is included analytically. These stem from elsewhere but serve as circumferences related to the close analysis and the actual site of engagement: the concepts of historical body and a broader societal discursive framing are, thus, embedded in the fine-tuned analysis of empirical data. This is done to closely explore a participant's perspective on the indeterminacies which generally define social practices. In the final chapter, the ground for the new proposed analytical perspective is discussed and recommendations are proposed.

Crucially, individuals with language and communication disorders are hindered in their display of meaning-making, even in co-construction of meaning with therapists and peers. The main conclusion of this contribution is that the effort to communicate is essentially the main challenge to an individual with a language or communication disorder. Notwithstanding this, indeterminacy is a present element in communication, even in deficit communication, if such can be said to exist outside a normative paradigm. Integrationism problematizes any linguistic assumptions or methods predicated on 'norms' or 'typicality'/'atypicality' of linguistic communication. Hence, from an integrational linguistic practice perspective, this book introduces a demythologized view on how all communication is communicative as it unfolds. This view accounts for a participants' perspective. In everyday life, participants display emotion, enter into arguments, and claim their unfulfilled wishes even when production is their main challenge. Apparently inert participants produce categories of competing discourses in interaction not because of their language and communication disorders or because of a lack of understanding the categories applied by peers. Cognitively, this would be highly devaluing of individuals. Empirically, it is demonstrated that persons seemingly engage in efforts far beyond their apparent abilities. This may point to the fact that to communicate matters to them regardless of the burden it is to perform it. Therefore, this monograph can be said to offer a new contribution to the field as it speaks against the frequently applied concepts of theory of mind and atypical interaction in the study of language and communication disorders (LCDs). As this book suggests, taking a practice stance on discourse in communication is part of the process of conveying this new analytical approach.

The book does not intend to provide a completely unfolded version of this view, nor a complete description of the implications of such a view. Therefore, it will not propose a model for a new analytical perspective but modestly draw the outline explaining the background for it. The aim of this study is, however, important for several reasons. It shows the possibility of integrating a participant's perspective in the study of language and communication disorders by changing the presuppositions of language and communication common to the field from clinical approaches to ethnomethodological ones. By implementing an integrational linguistic practice perspective, the very concepts of language and communication are sought to be demythologized at a philosophical level. This implementation also adds to a new agenda in practice studies. Rather, this book's implementation of a new perspective demonstrates that the individuals communicating are engaged in this world in complex ways. On this ground, language and communication (disorders) should be revisited as phenomena at a final stage of the communication and practice turns.

Furthermore, this book contributes to improved peer understanding of the integrational proficiency (Harris 2009, p. 71) of individuals with communication deficiencies such as linguistic and cognitive impairments (Nielsen 2011, 2015). Organizational intervention (Nielsen 2015; Simmons-Mackie and Damico 2008; Wilkinson 2011) should draw more closely on the experienced understandings of the people communicating. This book also aids policy development and evaluation. Finally, QOL-assessment of the psychosocial consequences of ABI and aphasia should follow the standards of the International Classification of Functioning, Disability And Health (the ICF model) (WHO 2001, 2013). Importantly, local contexts should be taken into consideration with expert advice from researchers who can help align local context with the ICF-model.

References

Harris, R. (1981). *The language myth*. London: Duckworth.

Harris, R. (1996). *Signs, language and communication*. London: Routledge.

Harris, R. (1998). *Introduction to integrational linguistics*. Oxford: Pergamon.

Harris, R. (2009). *Integrationist notes and papers 2006–2008*. Gamlingay: Bright Pen.

Nicolini, D. (2009). Zooming in and out: Studying practices by switching theoretical lenses and trailing connections. *Organization Studies, 30*(12), 1391–1418.

Nielsen, C. (2011). Towards applied integrationism: Integrating autism in teaching and coaching sessions. *Language Sciences, 33*(4), 593–602.

Nielsen, C. (2015). Senhjerneskade i et forståelsesperspektiv. In S. Frimann, M. Sørensen, & H. Wentzer (Eds.), *Sammenhænge i sundhedskommunikation* (pp. 247–281). Aalborg: Aalborg Universitetsforlag.

Simmons-Mackie, N., & Damico, J. (2008). Exposed and embedded corrections in aphasia therapy: Issues of voice and identity. *International Journal of Language & Communication Disorders, 43*(1), 5–17.

Wilkinson, R. (2011). Changing interactional behavior: Using conversation analysis in intervention programmes for aphasic conversation. In C. Antaki (Ed.), *Applied conversation analysis: Intervention and change in institutional talk* (pp. 32–53). Basingstoke: Palgrave Macmillan.

World Health Organization. (2001). *The international classification of functioning, disability and health* (ICF). Geneva: WHO.

World Health Organization. (2013). *How to use the ICF: A practical manual for using the international classification of functioning, disability and health* (ICF, 2013 ed.). Geneva: WHO.

CHAPTER 2

Language and Communication—The Contexualized and "Person-Centered" Nature of Linguistic and Communicative Action

Abstract The integrational perspective introduced in this chapter is concerned with a broader concept of communication, both implicit and explicit. This chapter sets the scene for this book's diffractive enrichment of combining an integrational linguistic approach and a Practice theory approach to language and communication, including the methodology of ethnomethodology and conversation analysis. The ontological similarities and incompatibilities of this combination are discussed throughout the book. Despite the presence of ontological divergences, in order to operate on an interdisciplinary ground, the transcript practice, the presuppositions, and the methodology of ethnomethodology and conversation analysis are integrated complementarily as they afford data retrieval and enrich the analysis and its discussions instrumentally. Lay-strategies for obtaining knowledge on communication and language are contrasted with expert linguists' strategies.

Keywords Conversation analysis · Integrational linguistics Practice theory · Practice studies · Lay-oriented strategies

© The Author(s) 2018   7
C. M. B. Klemmensen, *Integrating the Participants' Perspective in the Study of Language and Communication Disorders*,
https://doi.org/10.1007/978-3-319-78634-6_2

NEW HORIZONS IN THE STUDY OF LANGUAGE AND COMMUNICATION

Positioning Integrational Linguistics

This chapter and the ones that follow offer an introduction to the basics of the concept of *radical indeterminacy*: a term and concept conveyed by the founding father of IL and integrationism, Roy Harris. This book limits its investigation to the distinct application of radical indeterminacy as a psychosocial applied linguistic concept. Other approaches to radical indeterminacy are, therefore, not included (Blackman and Venn 2010). The theoretical contribution of this book reviews IL in relation to interaction and practice studies. No thorough account for applied IL in relation to interaction studies and practice studies currently exists. In addition, an extensive, descriptive account for the broad sense of "communication situation" within the IL discourse is missing. The aim of this chapter is to offer a framework to bring the reader closer to an understanding of the ontology of IL, and radical indeterminacy and its prerequisites, which are central to an integrational practice perspective.

It has been claimed by integrationists, and by Harris himself, that the basis of IL is radically different from traditional linguistics and the language sciences (see for instance, Love 2004; Damm 2008; Duncker 2011; Pablé 2011; Orman 2017; Toolan 1996; www.harris.com; www.integrationists.com). Therefore, integrationism has, for decades, stood back to back with the rest of applied linguistics and studies in pragmatics (see for instance, Lund 2012; Hutton 2016). It may be claimed that integrationism is seldom a useful perspective in language-disorder studies. This author argues that IL may be considered a specialized inquiry into language within the language sciences.

The Functions of Language

Historically, the functions of language in social interaction were studied by Bronislaw Malinowski and further elaborated by Roman Jakobson in the early twentieth century, well before the pragmatic approach to language became a general agenda in the language sciences. Malinowski's ethnography uncovered the importance of context by reference to the experience of customs and community practices necessary to understand the determinacy of linguistic manifestations. Language and semiotic units were not to be understood as mere representations but as the actual habits and actions constituting a community (Malinowski 1923). While addressing the question of style, Jakobson (1960) introduced his model of communication, which includes Malinowski's concept of *context* (Senft 2009, p. 227). The message is at the center of Jakobson's model surrounded by context. In contrast, the mathematical theory of communication of Claude Shannon and Warren Weavers (1969) is based on the idea of transmission of information, where the only contexts included are noise and disturbances. The mathematical model gave rise to a dominant cognitivist approach in the language sciences known as computation. The transmission term advocates the idea that signs and symbols are being transmitted through a process of physical and mental coding and *decoding* (Reddy 1979, p. 303). However, all of the above somehow draw ontologically on structuralism, which is encapsulated in Saussure's idea of signs as representations for "something else." An integrational strand emphasizes that "signs are not either linguistic or nonlinguistic: They are crucially the result of a sign-maker's *contextualization*. In other words, the sign-maker makes something into a sign according to his or her contingent needs" (Pablé 2013, p. 96). Therefore, IL may be argued to have affinity towards a theory of action rather than language and communication. Accordingly, context is substantiated in IL and attributed to persons in the process of sign-making rather than to the settings or to the surroundings of language and communication taking place as in the case of earlier models of language and communication, which mainly aim to define linguistic determinacy.

A Hint from the Data

To grasp the importance of introducing and applying the alternative integrational theory of language and communication in the study of Language and Communication Disorders (LCDs), a short introduction to the data analyzed in this book is necessary. The topic of this book is aphasia and Acquired Brain Injury (ABI). Long-term engagement with gathering and analyzing ethnographic video data recorded at a care center has led this author to peculiar observations of everyday interactions between impaired individuals and their occupational therapists. Regardless of local inclusion policies, exclusion of impaired individuals recurs in interaction. Individuals with aphasia and ABI demonstrate communicational proficiencies far beyond their diagnoses, yet, they are often corrected, resulting in their resignation from dialogues. Rather than engaging with the strictly therapeutic side of brain injury, this study focuses more broadly on the interactions observed. In particular, it draws on observations of the supposedly impaired individuals in different situations. These have proved to be so diverse and to reach far beyond the presumed abilities of the individuals, that this author's primary concern has become to describe the non-normativity of the interactions observed and analyzed.

For instance, how could it be explained that the ambient character of therapeutic situations is phatic in linguistic style and, unfavorably, results in resignation rather than interactive participation (Nielsen 2015)? Contrastingly, non-therapeutic situations arise within the frame of therapy all the time, and are oriented quite differently by the individuals, both linguistically and interactionally.

These counterpointing discrepancies in the ability to participate cannot be explained by theories of signs alone. Nor can they be explained by the physiological and cognitive impairment. Nor can they be thoroughly explained in the paradigm of performative theories. A new take is, therefore, to develop a theory of *circumstantial proficiency*. It seems that rather than prerequisites such as predicted and inherent "abilities," it is the situations themselves and what is at stake communicatively that guide participation abilities When proficiency is studied in relation to circumstantial factors, then meaning-making is at the center of the analysis and studied as processual.

Demonstrably, there are incentives for the individuals to be able to act. In short, determinacy is not predefined but circumstantial. This take applies both to an EMCA perspective and a CA perspective (Garfinkel 1967; Heritage 1984; Sacks et al. 1974), an IL perspective as well as to a PT perspective (Harris 1996, 1998; Schatzki 2002). Therefore, an exploration of the pairing of an EMCA perspective, an applied IL perspective, and a PT perspective is sought for the first time. However, an IL perspective is introduced with a heavier weight of interest for two reasons. First, the ontology of IL differs from the ontology of EMCA regarding presuppositions of orderliness of situated social order. Second, it offers an unexplored conceptual framework for approaching an individual's strategies as individually creative rather than uniquely programmatic and ordered by shared methods. It is this author's belief that the ontology of

IL is ontologically compatible with PT (Schatzki 2002), which will be introduced at the beginning of Chapter 5.

Introducing Important Peer Positions

Generally, studies in social interaction rely on ontologies of communication and action in contexts. Current positions within the interaction research field and IL have much in common, though they diverge in the basic assumption of signs and their interpretation. Traditionally, this divergence opposes integrationism to segregationalism, or structuralism-based assumptions, according to a Harrisian integrational position (Fleming 1995, 1997). In traditional studies in CA, interaction and understanding have been widely covered, starting from the early days of the field (Sacks et al. 1974). The aim of CA is to understand the participants' perspective, which is noticeably different from traditional discourse analysis. Traditional discourse analysis frames concepts, for instance speech acts, which are prerequisites for analysis. CA builds upon the grounds of an analytical strategy, relying on recordings (tape, digital sound, or video recordings), which are processed into micro-transcripts demonstrating speech: pronounced words, sighing, micro-linguistic feedback, and gesturing. These traces of social interaction are interpreted with a "*proof-procedure*," which serves as the scientific validation of the CA analyst's seemingly correct and refutable interpretation of individuals' "displays" of understanding in conversations (Sacks et al. 1974, p. 729). This book, however, seeks to challenge the concept of proof-proceduring as the only scientifically possible validation and refutable interpretation of persons' understandings.

Essentially, integrationists are interested in how people go about integrating, in line with how CA analysts are interested in how people go about conducting everyday life in various settings. However, the applied integrational perspective relies on its own principles and on its own ontology of a lay-oriented language approach, which lies closer to the approach of PT and practice studies than to CA. This perspective will continue to be unfolded and discussed throughout the book.

A Mixed Friendship: Integrational Linguistics and Conversation Analysis

Different perspectives on IL described within the language sciences have so far discussed a theoretical perspective starting from Harris's book *The Language Myth* (1981), which provocatively stated a "myth theory" (Linell 2005, p. 30) that Harris claims is the object of study in traditional linguistics. However, to this day, no thorough account combining the insights of IL with studies in everyday practices exists (Fleming 1997). Nor is there an account of how to operate analytically on the grounds of the broad sense of a "communication situation" formulated within the IL discourse. A broader sense of the analytical situation challenges several applied linguistic approaches, including the programmatic CA procedures of proof-finding in local context (Sacks et al. 1974). However, this point has been highlighted and demonstrated as a distinguishing feature of an IL perspective on several occasions (Fleming 1995, 1997; Taylor 1982). Within the current EMCA community, there are ongoing discussions on how narrowly or broadly the tools from CA ought to be interpreted. The journal *Discourse Studies* (2016) dedicated a special issue to discuss CA's proof-procedure as temporal fixing of determinacy versus John Heritage's extensive work on epistemic engine markers (such as "oh") as regular markers, which provide determinacy for changes of states in conversations. In sum, proof-procedure is still at the heart of CA and determines its analytical perspective.

A New Kind of Integrational Linguistics

The traditions for applied integrationism are rather narrow (Duncker 2011; Fleming 1997). The Hong Kong group of contemporary integrationists has taken a stance on data, which, in this author's opinion, is rather theory-based (Pablé and Hutton 2015). In an integrational perspective, the stance on data has contributed to building upon an applied integrationism. However, the practical application of the theoretical perspective needs still to be investigated further, since suggestions end up entangled in a language-philosophical discussion rather than in hands-on analyses (Pablé and Hutton 2015).

Seemingly, traditional integrationists and contemporary integrationists who seek a practical application continue to agree on the claim that the ontology of "integrationism" is radical and different from that of traditional language science. This claim may be considered troublesome since, for decades, IL has been regarded a mere negation of the language sciences and linguistics. Therefore, this author argues that IL should be considered differently: a specialized, but not radical, perspective within the range of perspectives in the language sciences. On this basis this book will argue that IL can be applied in analysis of the practice of meaning.

Staying true to integrationism, communication is approached as processual practices of meaning in line with a CA approach rather than as a decoding of meaning: the common, contrasting, structuralism-based assumption about the activity of communication. However, indeterminacy plays an important part, ontologically, in separating an integrational perspective from a pure CA-approach. Whereas CA aims at orientations towards temporal determinacy, the integrationist aims at uncovering understanding as something more than displays in local contexts. The integrationist investigates communication processes as human states of being and human modes of action necessary for survival (Harris 1996, pp. 63–78; 1998, p. 29).

INTRODUCTION TO APPLIED INTEGRATIONISM

Roy Harris's notion of *integrational semiology* (Harris 1996, p. 154) has been discussed in various branches of the language sciences discipline. Only lately has it been taken seriously and applied in empirical studies (see for instance, Damm 2016; Davis 2001; Duncker 2011; Conrad 2011; Pablé and Hutton 2015; Nielsen 2011; Worsøe 2014). Namely, applied linguistics and pragmatic studies with a focus on aspects of communication have taken an interest in an IL ontology and integrationism as an applied theoretical perspective, and contemporary integrationists are preoccupied with further exploring the theoretical implications of IL (Pablé 2017). For instance, radical indeterminacy in language is unfolded as demonstrable indeterminacy in a person's understanding of the stream of consciousness, drawing on the personal anecdote as data. Hence, indeterminacy is enhanced and explored as a broadening advantage of the theory (Orman 2017). Yet, three key notions in IL have not been defined for analysis, essential if IL is to be applied. The following three concepts distinctly attend IL analytically, in this author's perception:

1. The broadly defined sense of communication situation.
2. The notion of contextualization.
3. The principle of *cotemporality*.

Earlier attempts to distinguish integrationism from EMCA and CA have demonstrated the pros and cons of operating on a combined basis (Fleming 1995; Hutton 2008; Taylor 2008). The strong use of sequentiality in CA versus contextualization and cotemporality in IL is compared and discussed. This book will illustrate attempts is to apply integrationism as an analytical practice. It will remain no secret that this is an attempt to synthesize integrationism with the tools of CA and EMCA.

A New Introduction to Harris' Semiotics

Many brilliant scholars have introduced Harris's semiotics in various contexts with the aim of communicating its theoretical aspects and their discrepancies with traditional linguistics and the philosophy of language (Love 2004, 2007; Pablé 2010; Taylor 2008; Toolan 1996, 2008). This introduction is short and different as it focuses solely on the aspects of the Harrisian semiotics which apply to practice studies as a point of departure.

To summarize, four principles can be drawn from the above very short—but core—understanding of Harris's semiotics:

1. Signs are made in certain, actual communication situations.
2. Signs are unique.
3. No process of communication is without context.
4. Communication is processual and dynamic by nature.

Accordingly, an integrational semiology is based upon the notion that a sign is not autonomous but integrated into the situation in which it occurs. Whoever engages in the understanding of any sign, so to speak, by merely engaging or identifying it, applies a form of agency which, in Harris's terms, is best described as "integrational proficiency" (Harris 1996, p. 154).

The above IL sign axioms have been criticized by Lund (2012) as insufficient to meet the criteria of "signhood" (Lund 2012, p. 4). Lund claims to refute Harris's central theses by examining them rhetorically. He offers a summary of central themes in Harris's semiotics, primarily targeted towards linguists, confirming the orthodox premises in traditional linguistics.

Harris's own central claim is that "signs are not given to us by Nature" (Harris 2009b, p. 87) but need to be continuously created by us. Therefore, signs articulate the complexity of our own situation and "their creation is itself the creation of knowledge, and, more importantly, the creation of untold possibilities for its further expansion" (Harris 2009b, p. 87). This claim is of interest to the present project since it is relevant to a practice approach as the persons communicating, their actions, and their agency are the point of departure for a new applied integrationism. In the analysis of LCDs, biomechanical abilities are pre-requisites which afford a necessity for an analytical focus on multimo-dality rather than on language and linguistics (Harris 1998; Thibault 2007). Since the persons communicating are at the center of the analysis, a broad definition of the notion of "communication situation" is needed, as situations are experienced differently by each one of us (Harris 1996, 1998, 2009a).

Harris defines communication processes as governed by a set of indi-vidually determined factors. Famously, he proposes three levels of fac-tors: biomechanical, macrosocial, and circumstantial (Harris 1998, p. 29; Harris 2009a, pp. 75–76), which determine a communication situation. He defines communication situations as governed by a set of individually determined factors. These are to be understood as follows.

Biomechanical Factors
Biomechanical factors are, for example, normal neurophysiological abil-ities to communicate, to simply perceive the sound of talk, or it may be having a disorder and not being able to speak or pronounce certain words.

Macrosocial Factors
Macrosocial factors are matters such as understanding the same lan-guage, knowing social game rules, being polite, having humor, and knowing how to perform social common practices such as not showing up late for an appointment.

Circumstantial Factors
As an example of a circumstantial factor, Harris points to a story where a friend has had a car accident on his way to church and therefore has not shown up to the wedding. This circumstantial factor would overrule the

macrosocial factor that one should not show up late for appointments (Harris 2009a, p. 76).

Hierarchy of Factors
In theory, there is a hierarchy since circumstantial factors out rule or change the other factors' impact on meaning-making. Circumstantial factors are the more important ones since they point to situational-specific occurrences and thus control the need for making new meaning and provoke new understanding (Harris 2009a, p. 76).

Integrational Communication and Meaning

In *Introduction to Integrational Linguistics* (1998), Harris accounts for the situational anchoring of utterances (Harris 1998, p. 68):

> The integrationist treats meanings not as semantic units established in advance by a fixed code, but as values that arise in context out of particular communication situations. The participants assign these values as part of the integration of activities involved. It is in this sense that, for the integrationist, communication involves a constant making and re-making of meaning. It is intrinsic to the continuous creative process that our engagement with language is.

Following this, Harris's threefold characteristics are introduced to begin the conceptualization of an applied IL-inspired analysis of practices. First, meanings are processual and hereby dynamic, they are not preestablished; thus, signs and words cannot be meaningfully isolated from the situations in which they are produced. Second, meanings are results of modes that actual persons are in while they are doing something else, for instance, as they are trying to go about understanding something. Third, meanings are "provisional determinacy" (Harris 1998, p. 85) because understanding and contextualization are constant activities, which entail a constant dynamic (individual), person-centered production of meaning (Harris 1987, p. 7). According to Harris, we cannot meaningfully isolate signs, words, or persons who are engaged in understanding something.

In *Integrationist Notes and Papers 2006–2008*, Harris specifies that "(m)eanings are values conferred upon signs by their role in articulating the integration of activities. Signs are made this way," (Harris 2009a, p. 76). Meanings are, thus, regarded as produced by individuals in communication situations and persons do change their understanding all along communication, as demonstrated by ethnomethodologists (Goodwin 1979; Sacks 1984; Schegloff 1992).

Understandings can be demonstrated explicitly by producing a turn in a dialogue, and they can also be implicit. Whether understandings are explicit, interpretative, linguistic signs or implicit self-knowledge (Harris 2009b, p. 87), the communication situation applies to the total of persons, sign production, and situation, according to an IL perspective (Harris 1998, p. 68). Harris's theoretical semiotics investigated in *Signs, Language and Communication* (Harris 1996, pp. 63–78) describes communication processes broadly, including communication between natural phenomena and humans. However, this study is limited to the study of interaction between humans and humans, and their use of objects in the material setting.

An Alternative Theorizing on Language and Communication

The benefits of IL and its potential analytical perspective are twofold. First, it is creating an outline for the possible application of an ethnomethodological theorizing on language and communication, based on an integrational ontology stating that language is indeterminate in the sense that indexicality and approximation in meaning is uniquely individual rather than uniquely social (Harris 1987, p. 7). This applies to the integrationist as opposed to CA assumptions. Second, it is developing a potential methodology for analysis based on new basic assumptions regarding signs and meaning.

TRADITIONAL COUNTER-POSITIONS

Inherent Meaning in Language

In a structuralist view, language users pick meanings from the representational historical body of language and meaning. However, questions about *whose* perception and experience it might be are nowhere addressed in structuralism. Crucially, the question of agency is central to the integrationist position on signs and meaning. In the structuralism-based paradigm, agency is addressed only syntactically as the subject of a sentence. Therefore, content has nothing to do with real-life situations.

Objectivized Content in Linguistic Representations

In structuralism, content (the signified) has the status of a reflection of some*thing else*, which is what ascribes content as inherent to language. Moreover, it objectivizes meaning, as structuralism assumes that the signification is a reflected phenomenon arbitrarily encapsulated in a sign. In this view, content is attached to language and not to actions. Signification is derived from its linguistic representation. This heritage from Saussure's theory of signs is based on distinguishing the "signifier" from the "signified," yet representation and meaning are assumed to be present in the very representation: the sign.

Signs, Language, and Communication

Signs do not exist as predetermined items in a system of "language."[1] Moreover, signification is not regarded as mirrored and reflected in a sign itself but considered "a function of the integrational proficiency which its identification and interpretation presuppose" (Harris 1996, p. 154). Content is meaning in the making, and signification exists only as part of somebody's communicative enterprise; signification, in its own right, is a direct experience of the perceivable meaningfulness of some*thing* to some*one*. It cannot preexist as a reflection of "a meaning" inherent in language, nor as a reflection of someone else's materially recorded experience.

Decompartmentalizing Linguistics

As demonstrated above, IL departs from both compartmentalized, traditional, general linguistics and from structuralism-based, modern, applied linguistics. These assume inherent systems of meaning in the traditional Saussurean sense. Consequently, the IL perspective is moving towards "a non-compartmentalized study of human interaction" (Pablé and Hutton 2015, p. 59). Epistemologically and ontologically, it suggests a radical sign theory and an alternative to traditional notions of meaning as something inherent in signs. Finally, it informs the established tradition in modern applied linguistics with an important supplement.

The Epistemology of the IL-Inspired Analysis

Analyses carried out with an IL inspired approach to the study of language and communication alter the status of observable units and the interpretation of their content. For instance, the study of dialogue dynamics in modern applied linguistics draws on presuppositions of orderliness and normativity in language use, thus pointing to a traditional framework. The starting point for the development of an IL-inspired methodology is the integration of theories of IL, the workings of language and communication, and considering and describing the mythical assumption-based framework of structuralism which still dominates basic beliefs about the signification of displays in EMCA (Harris 1996, 1998; Toolan 1996; Fleming 1995; Pablé and Hutton 2015).

A Folk Science of Signs and Communication

Let us consider sign production and sign interpretation as persons' understandings. Several accounts of interaction patterns exist from EMCA, but we know very little about what is actually understood by the individuals in interaction, though we all possess lay-knowledge and can easily account for our understandings. As demonstrated by Linda Svenstrup (2002, 2008), individuals, when confronted with the analyst's results of their interactions and situated understandings, often reply that the analytical result was not what the individual was trying to say nor even close to his or her own interpretation of the situation and the sequence analyzed. This places us with a methodological challenge when discrepancies occur between individuals' experienced world and the experts' data representations of the experiences of the individuals. The first step towards incorporating IL in the science of languages is to thus position IL as a folk science, a folkloristic interaction perspective, so to say (Nielsen and Solvang 2012). This perspective is rather different from a more philosophical perspective stated earlier by integrationists (Pablé 2010 2017; Love 2007). The proposition of an analytical approach takes IL in a new and different direction when aligning it with practice studies. This will be expanded upon in the following section, and in Chapters 4, 5, and 6.

BUILDING ON AN INTEGRATIONAL PRACTICE PERSPECTIVE

The Practice Turn

The recent "practice turn" (Reckwitz 2002) has a focus on everyday emergent practices. A theoretical lens emphasizes the emergent nature of everyday, organizational, social life, and routines in which meanings, bodies, minds, things, knowledge, discourses, structures, agency, identities, and other entities or processes are accomplished and momentarily fixed. Academically, the practice turn gains terrain because it is so useful. Practices may be mapped and described in order to assess, improve, or change practice procedures (Nicolini 2012; Clarke 2005; Scollon and Scollon 2004). Practice research is setting the research agenda out of a need to grasp the complexity of everyday practice. Taking a practice stance allows for a flexible approach. It has the flux property of changing foci ongoingly during the research process as insight is gained (Scollon and Scollon 2004). Drawing on the works of Andreas Reckwitz (2002), Ron Scollon and Suzie Scollon (2004), Adele Clarke (2005), Theodore Schatzki (2002), Davide Nicolini (2009, 2012), and the recent practice anthology of Anders Horsbøl and Pirkko Raudaskoski (2016), to name the major contributors that are indebted, practices practiced are what define the practice approach to LCDs applied in this book.

The expanding boundary of the study of LCDs are in part a consequence of a more general growing interest in interdisciplinary studies within applied linguistics and interaction studies, leading towards an applied practice perspective. This upcoming focal area of investigating "how it is done out there in the field" owes much of its interest to the influence and traditions of EMCA. The studies of conversation and conversational settings of Harvey Sacks and Emanuel Schegloff gave Charles Goodwin and Ray Wilkinson the tools to carry out their pioneering studies in LCDs and speech therapy (see for instance, Goodwin 2003; Wilkinson 2011). Charles Goodwin (1995, p. 235) switched focus from linguistic interpretation to the interpretation of activities in his first studies of an aphasic man. Moreover, there has been a more general interest and request to make embodied talk and materiality relevant both in pioneering multimodal and video analysis, as demonstrated extensively by Goodwin (see Goodwin 2010; Goodwin et al. 2012).

Inquiry into LCDs through video observation called for a need for multimodal transcripts where inquiry is allowed to approach the bodily expressions, such as emotions, conveyed towards the objects present or associated (Goodwin et al. 2012; James 1950, pp. 442–485). This turn, later labeled CA, developed a whole new and broader concept of context and contextual configurations and participatory analysis (e.g. Goodwin 2000; Wilkinson 2011), which differed from traditional CA and EM studies. The analytical approach in the study of LCDs which has been developed in the augmented version of the CA tradition, multimodal interaction analysis, is much more concerned with room setting, material objects, multimodality, and communicational logistics and routines than it is with tracking mere language as in the traditional linguistic sense. Suddenly, the individual with impairment is no longer being scrutinized, but the surrounding responses to his or her contributions and presence form part of the interpretive repertoire, elements of the local institutional setting are included, and situated discourses are identified. Objects in use are considered important elements, and the distribution and logistics of language, minds, and bodies may account for situated configurations of coordination and discursive positioning.

Practice Theory—A Rapidly Expanding Field

Within its own arena, practice research itself is a rapidly expanding field. It includes various focal areas of interest and a variety of traditions, ranging from business communication (Nicolini 2012; Alvesson and Sköldberg 2018), to theoretical discourse studies (Angermuller 2013; Angermuller et al. 2014), to media analysis (Cooren 2015), to environmental studies, and the studies of disappearing languages (Scollon and Scollon 2004, 2007), technical system operation and maintenance, aphasia (Goodwin 1995, 2003; Wilkinson 2011), and researching health communication (Sarangi 2007). The aim is to study individuals who are routinely applying their everyday and professional knowledge to combine their actions with others in order to perform their everyday life or their profession, such as technical system maintenance, identity, or corporate identity.

Tools in Practice Research

Ron Scollon and Suzie Scollon offer a unique tool to grasp the object of practice studies independent of whichever area one is studying in the various fields within practice studies. The first steps in their approach, nexus analysis, introduces a frame and methodology to navigate, identify, and map practices (Scollon and Scollon 2004, 2007, 2009).

Placing the study of LCDs and speech therapy within the field of practice studies allows for a whole new and unique analytical perspective, which this book further develops. Thereby, the present approach to a new study of LCDs is placed far from traditional applied linguistics. This approach differs uniquely from the objects studied in traditional linguistics and interaction studies in the EM tradition, which deals with language, such as talk and utterances, and which apply and operate analytical concepts, such as local context. When applying the approaches of Goodwin and Wilkinson in a practice studies perspective rather than an EM perspective, then the lives lived with LCDs are approached from a new angle.

NOTE

1. In 1996, Roy Harris published *Signs, Language and Communication: Integrational and Segregational Approaches*. The book distinguishes IL from other theories of language and communication by pointing to the structuralism-based (segregational) presuppositions in basically all other sign theories.

REFERENCES

Alvesson, M., & Sköldbjerg. (2018). *Reflexive methodology* (2nd ed.). Thousand Oaks, CA: Sage.

Angermuller, J. (2013). How to become an academic philosopher: Academic discourse as a multileveled positioning practice. *Sociología Histórica, 2*, 263–289.

Angermuller, J., Maingueneau, D., & Wodak, R. (Eds.). (2014). *Main currents in theory and analysis*. Amsterdam: John Benjamins.

Blackmann, L., & Venn, C. (2010). Affect. *Body and Society, 16*(1), 7–28.

Clarke, A. (2005). *Situational analysis: Grounded theory after the postmodern turn*. Thousand Oaks, CA: Sage.

Conrad, C. (2011). *Forståelseshandlingen: En empirisk afprøvet teori om narrativ forståelse som situeret betydning i dannelse*. PhD dissertation, Københavns Universitet, København.

Cooren, F. (2015). In medias res: Communication, existence, and materiality. *Communication Research and Practice, 1*(4), 307–321.

Damm, B. (2008). Hvad er sprog i virkeligheden? *Nydanske Sprogstudier, 36*, 151–172.

Damm, B. (2016). *Sproglig betydningsdannelse i teori og praksis: En teoretisk og empirisk videreudvikling af det integrerede sprogsyn.* PhD dissertation, Københavns Universitet, København.

Davis, H. (2001). *Words: An integrational approach.* Richmond, Surrey: Curzon Press.

Discourse Studies. (2016). Special issue: The epistemics of epistemics, *18*(5).

Duncker, D. (2011). On the empirical challenge to integrational studies in language. *Language Sciences, 33*(4), 533–543.

Fleming, D. (1995). The search for an integrational account of language: Roy Harris and conversation analysis. *Language Sciences, 17*(1), 73–98.

Fleming, D. (1997). Is ethnomethodological conversation analysis an "integrational" account of language? In G. Wolf & N. Love (Eds.), *Linguistics inside out* (pp. 182–207). Amsterdam: John Benjamins.

Garfinkel, H. (1967). Studies of the routine grounds of everyday activities. In G. Psathas (Ed.), *Studies in ethnomethodology* (pp. 35–75). Cambridge: Polity Press.

Goodwin, C. (1979). The interactive construction of a sentence in natural conversation. In G. Psathas (Ed.), *Studies in ethnomethodology* (pp. 12–97). Cambridge: Polity Press.

Goodwin, C. (1995). Co-constructing meaning in conversation with an aphasic man. *Research on Language and Social Interaction, 28*(3), 233–260.

Goodwin, C. (2000). Action and embodiment within human interaction. *Journal of Pragmatics, 32*, 1489–1522.

Goodwin, C. (2003). Conversational frameworks for the accomplishment of meaning in aphasia. In C. Goodwin (Ed.), *Conversation and brain damage* (pp. 90–116). Oxford: Oxford University Press.

Goodwin, C. (2010). Multimodality in human interaction. *Calidoscópio, 8*(2), 85–98.

Goodwin, M., Cekaite, A., & Goodwin, C. (2012). Emotion as stance. In A. Peräkylä & M. Sorjonen (Eds.), *Emotion in interaction* (pp. 16–41). Oxford: Oxford University Press.

Harris, R. (1981). *The language myth.* London: Duckworth.

Harris, R. (1987). *The language machine.* Ithaca, NY: Cornell University Press.

Harris, R. (1996). *Signs, language and communication.* London: Routledge.

Harris, R. (1998). *Introduction to integrational linguistics.* Oxford: Pergamon.

Harris, R. (2009a). *Integrationist notes and papers 2006–2008.* Gamlingay: Bright Pen.

Harris, R. (2009b). *After epistemology.* Gamlingay: Bright Pen.

Heritage, J. (1984). *Garfinkel and ethnomethodology.* Oxford: Basil Blackwell.

Horsbøl, A., & Raudaskoski, P. (Eds.). (2016). *Diskurs og praksis: Teori, metode og analyse.* København: Samfundslitteratur.

Hutton, C. (2008). Meaning and the principle of linearity. In R. Harris & G. Wolf (Eds.), *Integrational linguistics: A first reader* (pp. 126–142). Bingley: Emerald Group Publishing Limited.

Hutton, C. (2016). The impossible dream? Reflections on the intellectual journey of Roy Harris (1913–2015). *Language and History, 59*(1), 79–84.

Jakobson, R. (1987). Linguistics and poetics. In K. Pomorska & S. Rudy (Eds.), *Language in literature* (pp. 62–94). Cambridge, MA: Harvard University Press (Origin. 1960).

James, W. (1950). *The principles of psychology* (Vol. 2). Cambridge, MA: Harvard University Press (Origin. 1890).

Linell, P. (2005). *The written language bias.* Abingdon: Routledge.

Love, N. (2004). Cognition and the language myth. Distributed cognition and integrational linguistics. *Language Sciences, 26*(6), 525–544.

Love, N. (2007). Are languages digital codes? *Language Sciences, 29*(5), 690–709.

Lund, S. (2012). On professor Harris's "integrational turn" in linguistics. *RASK, 35*(1), 3–42.

Malinowski, B. (1923). The problem of meaning in primitive language. In C. Ogden & I. Richards (Eds.), *The meaning of meaning: A study of the influence of language upon thought and of the science of symbolism* (pp. 296–325). San Diego: Harcourt, Brace and World.

Nicolini, D. (2009). Zooming in and out: Studying practices by switching theoretical lenses and trailing connections. *Organization Studies, 30*(12), 1391–1418.

Nicolini, D. (2012). *Practice theory, work, and organization: An introduction.* Oxford: Oxford University Press.

Nielsen, C. (2011). Towards applied integrationism: Integrating autism in teaching and coaching sessions. *Language Sciences, 33*(4), 593–602.

Nielsen, C. (Speaker), & Solvang, H. (Producer). (2012, May 31). Sprogpsykologi: Et eller andet med sprog [radio show episode]. In *Sproglaboratoriet.* København: Danmarks Radio.

Nielsen, C. (2015). Senhjerneskade i et forståelsesperspektiv. In S. Frimann, M. Sørensen, & H. Wentzer (Eds.), *Sammenhænge i sundhedskommunikation* (pp. 247–281). Aalborg: Aalborg Universitetsforlag.

Orman, J. (2017). Indeterminacy in sociolinguistics and integrationist theory. In A. Pablé (Ed.), *Critical humanist perspectives: The integrational turn in philosophy of language and communication* (pp. 96–113). London: Routledge.

Pablé, A. (2010). Language, knowledge and reality: The integrationist on name variation. *Language & Communication, 30*(2), 109–122.

Pablé, A. (2011). Integrating the "real". *Language Sciences, 33*(1), 20–29.

Pablé, A. (2013). Integrating Rorty and (social) constructivism: A view from a Harrisian semiology. *Social Epistemology, 29*(1), 95–117.

Pablé, A. (Ed.). (2017). *Critical humanist perspectives: The integrational turn in philosophy of language*. London: Routledge.

Pablé, A., & Hutton, C. (2015). *Signs, meaning and experience*. Berlin: De Gruyter Mouton.

Reckwitz, A. (2002). Towards a theory of social practices: A development in culturalist theorizing. *European Journal of Social Theory, 5*(2), 243–263.

Reddy, M. J. (1979). The conduit metaphor: A case of conflict metaphor in our language about our language. In A. Ortony (Ed.), *Metaphor and thought* (pp. 284–324). Cambridge: Cambridge University Press.

Sacks, H. (1984). On doing "being ordinary". In J. Atkinson & J. Heritage (Eds.), *Structures of social action: Studies in conversation analysis* (pp. 413–429). Cambridge: Cambridge University Press.

Sacks, H., Schegloff, E., & Jefferson, G. (1974). A simplest systematics for the organization of turn-taking for conversation. *Language, 50*(4), 696–735.

Sarangi, S. (2007). The anatomy of interpretation: Coming to terms with the analyst's paradox in professional discourse studies. *Text and Talk, 27*(5/6), 567–584.

Schatzki, T. (2002). *The site of the social: A philosophical account of the constitution of social life and change*. University Park: Pennsylvania State University Press.

Schegloff, E. (1992). Repair after next turn: The last structurally provided defense of intersubjectivity in conversation. *American Journal of Sociology, 97*(5), 1295–1345.

Scollon, R., & Scollon, S. W. (2004). *Discourse and the emerging internet*. London: Routledge.

Scollon, R., & Scollon, S. W. (2007). Nexus analysis: Refocusing ethnography on action. *Journal of Sociolinguistics, 11*(5), 608–625.

Scollon, S. W. (2009). Peak oil and climate change in a rural Alaskan community: A sketch of a nexus analysis. *Journal of Applied Linguistics, 6*(3), 357–378.

Senft, G. (2009). Phatic communion. In G. Senft, O. Östman & J. Verschueren (Eds.), *Culture and language use* (pp. 226–233). *Handbook of Pragmatics: Highlights 2*. Amsterdam: John Benjamins.

Shannon, C. & Weaver, W. (1969). *The mathematical theory of communication* (4th ed.). Chicago: The University of Illinois Press (Origin. 1945).

Svenstrup, L. (2002). Et signifikant perspektiv på samtalen: om sprogpsykologiske analyser af samtaler og analytiske konsekvenser af et sprogpsykologisk syn på sprog og kommunikation. Masters thesis, Institut for Almen og Anvendt Sprogvidenskab (unpublished), København.

Svenstrup, L. (2008). Sprogpsykologi. In L. Svenstrup, K. Risager, & N. Wille (Eds.), *Den sproglige verden* (pp. 28–65). Aarhus: Systime.

Taylor, T. (1982). *Discontinuity in conversational speech: An investigation of some theoretical problems and their analysis*. PhD dissertation, Trinity College, Oxford.

Taylor, T. (2008). Do you understand? In R. Harris & G. Wolf (Eds.), *Integrational linguistics: A first reader* (pp. 198–208). Bingley: Emerald Group Publishing Limited.

Toolan, M. (1996). *Total speech: An integrational linguistic approach to language.* Durham, NC: Duke University Press.

Toolan, M. (2008). A few words on telementation. In R. Harris & G. Wolf (Eds.), *Integrational linguistics: A first reader* (pp. 68–82). Bingley: Emerald Group Publishing Limited.

Wilkinson, R. (2011). Changing interactional behavior: Using conversation analysis in intervention programmes for aphasic conversation. In C. Antaki (Ed.), *Applied conversation analysis: Intervention and change in institutional talk* (pp. 32–53). Basingstoke: Palgrave Macmillan.

Worsøe, L. (2014). *Nye ord på nye måder: Nyorddannelse belyst fra et dynamisk sprog- og kognitionssyn.* PhD dissertation, Københavns Universitet, København.

CHAPTER 3

Language and Communication Disorders as an Area of Study

Abstract Traditionally, problems with language and communication have been approached through a discourse of disabledness or deficiency. In contract, this book explores and challenges this understanding, turning the spotlight on divergent discourses in current research in language and communication disorders (LCDs). Two cases are compared for this purpose: autism and aphasia. Studies in autism presuppose the mind to be an impersonal decoding machine. On the other hand, studies in aphasia presuppose the social to be the essence of human existence. In this view, co-construction of meaning and participation have replaced the individualist stance. In consequence, aphasia studies are enhancing a discourse of abledness while traditional autism studies are advocating a discourse of disabledness. Accordingly, explanation for the development in aphasia studies is sought.

Keywords Conditions for description · Metaphorical terminology Ontology · Clinical discourse · Everyday discourse

LANGUAGE AND COMMUNICATION DISORDERS

In recent years, the scope of the study of language and communication in the field of language and communication disorders (LCDs) has expanded beyond its origins in linguistics and interaction studies.

© The Author(s) 2018   27
C. M. B. Klemmensen, *Integrating the Participants' Perspective in the Study of Language and Communication Disorders*,
https://doi.org/10.1007/978-3-319-78634-6_3

It is, for instance, beginning to encompass interdisciplinary fields such as ethnographic medical studies, interdisciplinary discourse studies, and language psychology. It no longer necessarily involves a strict focus on either language or on language deficiency. Different areas of study have developed and carry different traditions. For instance, while the study of responselessness following autism largely draws on an individualist approach from developmental psychology with a sole focus on the individuals with autism, the study of aphasia following ABI has developed an analytical tradition, which largely includes and draws on ethnographical methodology and studies co-construction in participatory frameworks. These two counter-positions illustrate the diversity of contemporary research in language disorders. Further, they constitute two different narratives in modern studies of language disorders. One tells an individualist story of language disorders as an effect of mental disability, while the other tells a story based on social practice and co-operative meaning-making.

Increasingly, a strict, individualist clinical approach is becoming less popular as it is challenged by a social practice discourse (Gergen 2015). Overall, developmental factors in society and in medicine may help explain some of these new tendencies. To name a few, first, professional practitioners are looking for pragmatic solutions to practical problems in their everyday life. Second, contemporary welfare societies, at least in the Western culture, apply concepts such as patient-centeredness, patient safety, and holistic nursing. Third, due to the wide distribution of information on the Internet, individuals themselves increasingly explore knowledge about conditions and treatments. Furthermore, they are aware of an individual's right to complain over treatment and clinical assessment. As a result, relatives and peers participate far more in medical assessments than was the case in earlier times, when assessment pertained exclusively to the clinical experts. Therefore, in order to draw a fuller picture of the topography of the current field, it is important to point to the importance and the relevance of studying everyday life for several of the above reasons.

Understanding the Case of Linguistic Impairment

Linguistic impairment and brain damage are often associated. Brain injury, whether it was acquired at birth or later in life, traditionally has been regarded as a malfunction. It has been approached and understood as a biological deficit or as a cognitive disability. Whenever individuals have what most traditional frameworks label as communicational deficiencies, the analyses of communicational possibilities are primarily based on a cognitive model. This means that the focus is on processes and processing of the individual, where the individual is primarily observed isolated from his or her daily contexts. For instance, the research agenda in the field of autism has long been dominated by the research discourse (Nielsen 2011, 2013, p. 1). Several researchers now position themselves as critical towards strictly clinical approaches, which biologize human conditions in different fields in health communication (Brinkmann 2010, pp. 27–28). Health research now tends to call for a broader focus on social aspects.

Understanding Health-Related Disorders as Biologically Based

Regarding investigations of health matters, it is important to discuss the latent understanding of the theme or subject approached. Traditionally, disorders have been approached biologically, as mentioned above. This approach is grounded in a certain understanding of health and of the individual. A biological understanding of disorders in language and communication presupposes an array of interrelated processing in the individual. This view is closely related to a cognitivist view. Thus, language and communication deficiencies are perceived as bound to certain physiological dysfunctional bio-mechanisms or atypical neurological states. In this view, disorders are considered linked to certain damage to the functional system, which may include body, mind, and relations to other bodies and minds. For example, an inherent injury to the frontal lobes in the brain (considered an altered physiological basis) could cause a cognitive deficiency (an altered mental state), which ultimately leads to the diagnosis of an autism spectrum disorder (see for instance, Baron-Cohen 1995). In a biological interpretation of LCDs, the interrelated array of deficient functionalities defines this view: a damage to the frontal lobes which naturally affects the processing of perceptual input, which affects cognitive processing, which affects emotional response and bodily movement. In a bio-perspective, the damage is the very point of departure of a system breakdown which leads to states of cognitive deficiency. Finally, the idea of a stepwise process conceptualizes the bio-approach to deficiency in language and communication studies.

The Case of Autism

The bio-approach takes for granted that the deficit of linguistic and communicative response in individuals with autism is caused by an injury in the brain. Many discoveries in the case of autism have been conceptualized from this view. However, many interaction discourse studies of individuals with autism largely refute the strictly bio-based perspective applied to autism as the only way of approaching and treating the disorder scientifically (Korkiakangas et al. 2016; Rae and Ramey 2015; Sterponi 2004; Sterponi and de Kirby 2016; Leudar and Costall 2011; Björne 2007, to name several). These authors have all examined autism in everyday life. Together, they challenge dominant clinical descriptive practice by recording discrepancies in everyday behavior of individuals with autism, as opposed to the clinical descriptions that define their condition. Trouble sources in the interactional environment, for instance peer fashions of linguistic questioning and activity cueing, are given as much attention as the difficulties displayed by the individual with autism in isolation. In addition, supportive strategies for scaffolding interaction are being explored in the works of Laura Sterponi and John Rae. Notwithstanding, the major diagnostic manuals, the American Psychiatric Association's *Diagnostic and Statistical Manual of Mental Disorders*, fifth edition (DSM-5) (APA 2013) and the WHO's *International Statistical Classification of Diseases and Related Health Problems*, tenth revision (ICD-10) (WHO 2016), are solely based on the bio-perspective, as discussed by Nielsen (2013, pp. 2–4). The diagnostic criteria formulated in the DSM-5 as well as the descriptions in the ICD-10[1] draw on test situations from cognitive and developmental psychology and do not include the ever-increasing number of contemporary interaction studies refuting these tests (Nielsen 2013; Korkiakangas et al. 2016; Rae and Ramey 2015; Sterponi 2004; Sterponi and de Kirby 2016; Leudar and Costall 2011; Björne 2007). However, the terminology of the diagnostic manuals is of great medical importance regarding the provision of health and social care services to individuals. Services to individuals with severe LCDs are linked to the categorization of physical and cognitive impairment due to the array mechanism of the bio-perspective.

Traditionally, the discourse in autism research is strictly bio-based. The most frequently applied concept, mindblindness, is derived from a metaphorical conceptualization of how individuals with autism communicate and demonstrate participation through testing oral understanding and bodily orientation. The book *Mindblindness* by Baron-Cohen (1995) has played a founding role in establishing the theory of mind (ToM). ToM suggests that we have a theory working inside us when we are operating in everyday life and in the process of understanding others (Leslie 1987, pp. 412–426; Baron-Cohen et al. 1985, pp. 37–46). In *Mindblindness* (1995), autism is categorized as a neurodevelopmental cognitive disorder. It is described as an inability to operate a ToM properly. Basically, the concept presupposes that the individual with autism lacks decoding information and cannot, for instance, orient socially and coordinate with the actions of others because the "mindblind" cannot decode what others are thinking, feeling, and intending. Frith (2003) defines autism as an impairment of the mind derived from brain damage. Notwithstanding, Frith explains the enigma of autism as a lack of communicative competence in agreement with the DSM-5 definition of autism disorders (First et al. 2004, pp. 377–378; Frith 2003, p. 117). According to Baron-Cohen and Frith, language and communication are bio-based concepts: something is being processed incorrectly in the mind-machine resulting from brain damage. In this view, autism is a simple mind-dysfunction inhibiting individuals from appropriate participation in social life. By presupposing that the individual with autism lacks decoding information for operating a ToM, this metaphorical terminology claims that mind is a segregated concept.

However, in a functionalist view, deficiency is represented alongside the societal context of the pathological condition. This approach to considering health issues in a broader sense than the isolated bio-based perspective allows for a joint understanding, which is growing and becoming an established discourse. It is now being supported by the WHO. In conclusion, an individualist stance is claimed as central to explaining participation in the world. This idea in autism studies about the mind is derived from studying individuals with autism in a neuropsychological conceptualization of autism.

The Functionalist/Functioning Approach to Language and Communication Disorders

Overall, the WHO's conceptual framework for the ICF-model, liberates the individual from a potential burden of responsibility for his or her "disability" (WHO 2001, 2013). In addition, a functionalist understanding of LCDs takes point of departure in the above conceptual framework implicitly, as it is grounded in observations of everyday challenges to the individual. The interactional field research and inquiries into LCDs are notably unified. A recent special issue of the journal *Aphasiology* (2015) demonstrates and summarizes advances in the field, drawing on CA. This view allows for a functionalist study in both speech therapy and everyday settings, where pathologists and peers close to the individual with aphasia are studied with an analytic focus on the concept of repair in speech in interaction (Wilkinson 2015, p. 259). This research is carried out in CA-tradition. Indeed, this contemporary analytical perspective in the study of aphasia is more in alignment with the international recommendations from the WHO (2001, 2013, 2015) as it explicitly distinguishes the biological damage from participatory abilities in everyday life and in society. Internationally, the functionalist view is growing in popularity and is becoming a preferred approach in disability studies, as well; as at a more general level in professional health and social care. Regarding both the conceptual framework and the assessment of interventions, the WHO is trialing previous norms for practices, adding both to professional practices and to research. Ultimately, the idea of conceptualizing intervention standards worldwide can be discerned as an attempt to secure the well-being of individuals and the population at large by promoting a patient-centered awareness in society, including health research and professional practice.

The Lived Experience of Disabilities and Disorders

In an existentialist humanist perspective (Bøttcher and Dammeyer 2010, p. 30), personhood and the personal and peer-shared experience of the physiological, cognitive, and social sides of disabilities and disorders have great impact in explaining the many varieties of the lived experience. To phrase it differently, the "lived extent" of the clinical condition may differ immensely from person to person and from community to community. Aimee Mullins, star athlete and activist, is an individual who continuously explores the creative possibilities of missing legs. She may participate in the Paralympics and own twelve pairs of prosthetic legs, each suitable for different contexts, and enjoy this lived experience (http://www.ted.com/talks/aimee_mullins_prosthetic_aesthetics). Contrastingly, others with prosthetics may be sitting alone, isolated from friends, and may experience and suffer from social exclusion and depression as a consequence of missing limbs or ill-fitting prosthetics.

On the contrary, we must not overlook that identity cultures exist based on unique linguistic and communicational features. McIllvenny and Raudaskoski (1994), McIllvenny (1995) demonstrate this in interaction studies. They find that the interaction patterns in deaf societies cultivate unique discursive identity markers based on their supposed societal disability. The deaf define and consider themselves a community. Based on this, it is hard to claim that a unified perception of approaches to language disorders as such is detectable from one end of the LCDs scale to the other. Some groups may react quite differently even within the group, whilst a community such as the deaf practices a unique social community grounded in not hearing, sign language, and a locally founded common sense. In modern online fora, these findings are retrievable and easily validated in a plethora of chat-rooms focused on autism, acquired brain damage, and so on.

Towards a Practice Approach to Language and Communication Disorders

Drawing on Vygotsky, a dialectic understanding of disability and LCDs is an approach which considers disability and disorders inseparable from considering every person's psychology as cultural-historical phenomena (Bøttcher and Dammeyer 2010, p. 33). This view is closely linked to an IL approach to communication and language, as Vygotsky considers the importance of understanding the complex relationship between inner biological (biomechanical) and outer social (macrosocial) factors (Bøttcher and Dammeyer 2010, p. 33; Harris 1998, p. 29).

The Case of Aphasia

In the study of aphasia, current discourse identifies and maps this disorder as a matter of linguistic deficiency, categorizing it as an atypical mode of communication (Antaki and Wilkinson 2013). Furthermore, aphasia categorizes as memory problems, sensory disturbances, and other cognitive and physical impairments. Frequently, these features mean that the individual with impairment is limited communicatively. Limitations in communication make it difficult for an individual to engage with other people, and vice versa.

The presence of deficiencies and impairments in atypical modes of communication is a feature of a variety of language disorders; apart from aphasia, autism, Down syndrome, deafness, and various conditions of cognitive impairment, may be included. Antaki and Wilkinson (2013) label language disorders into categories of "atypical populations." The atypical populations are divided into three categories: the first embraces cases where cognition is intact but difficulties in speech and hearing may occur; the second contains cognitive impairments, such as those associated with autism and Down syndrome; the third includes atypical beliefs, cases where speech and language are intact but beliefs may cause disturbances and produce atypicalities, as in the cases of psychotic states and schizophrenia (Antaki and Wilkinson 2013, pp. 533–534). Aphasia is characterized by problems in the production of speech. Its two most common features are a lack of word retrieval (anomia) or disfluent aphasia (agrammatism or Broca's aphasia, typically from acquired brain injury).

CA is a preferred analytical approach to aphasic conversation (Antaki and Wilkinson 2013). In interaction studies, the study of communicative impairment, such as the case of aphasia, typically include a study, an investigation, and a demonstration of the person with impairment's initiative, sustenance, and termination of an interaction. Moreover, interaction studies explore and describe mechanisms of the co-construction of meaning on CA. The presuppositions of CA are based on communication's orderliness (Wilkinson 1999a, b). In addition, orderliness encompasses an organized, semiotic framework; the semiotic nature of signs and gesturing as well as the semiotic nature of enactment with the physical environment (Perkins 2003; Goodwin 2000, 2003b; Wilkinson et al. 2011). Three main collections account for this semiotic tradition and tendency (Goodwin 2003a; *Aphasiology* 1999, 2015). Notwithstanding, this assumption-based framework of CA points to a structuralist dominance in EMCA seen from an IL perspective drawing on the theoretical discussion in the previous chapter (Harris 1996, 1998; Toolan 1996; Fleming 1995; Love 2007; Pablé and Hutton 2015).

Methodologically, researchers are inevitably challenged by questions of the possible interpretation of interactional displays by the individual with impairment: how much the analyst attributes what is displayed or not displayed to the production time and the organization of repair may seem inactive and extended (Perkins 2003; Raudaskoski 2013). No one definitively knows how much to ascribe to intentional communication.

Moreover, no one holds the answer on how to manage comprehension deficiency.

At first sight, autism and aphasia are types of atypical communication that seem to have little in common; their clinical symptoms and neuro-atypicalities do diverge. However, the compensatory strategies used in interaction by the individuals affected by autism and aphasia after trauma have proved to be strikingly similar. First, in aphasic conversation the frequent occurrence of test questions (Simmons-Mackie and Damico 2008) has been given particularly close research attention. This phenomenon often occurs in institutional settings such as classrooms and in therapy. The teacher or therapist asks for information from the student or the aphasic, which s/he knows the answer to. Autism research has shown that persons with impaired communication abilities reject this practice as they treat it as unreal; resignation is the interactional consequence (Harris 2009; Nielsen 2011, 2015; Tammet 2006). Similarly, persons with aphasia react similarly when exposed to unreal practices such as treatment in occupational therapy (Raudaskoski 2013; Nielsen 2015). Furthermore, individuals with impairments like aphasia suffer from excessive other-initiated correction (Simmons-Mackie and Damico 2008). In conclusion, the practice of test questioning as the core activity in conversation may inhibit the inclusion of individuals with language disorders in interaction as it engenders inauthenticity. Authenticity is important to rehabilitate a person after trauma, as well as maintaining and developing personhood circumstantially. The opposite case of pretense gaming is in danger of disabling the person with impairment further.

Second, in studies on participating with language disorders, another area of attention is on repair organization and linguistic asymmetry in interaction (Goodwin 2003a). The interactional order and the organization of repair are studied in formal and informal settings with individuals who demonstrate limited competencies in speaking and comprehension. Explicit repair work is extensive in the case of aphasia, since aphasia is characterized by problems in the production of speech (Perkins 2003). Contrastingly, in autism research, repair work is more frequently implicit and is mainly uncovered in interviews and biographies (Tammet 2006; Nielsen 2011). In conclusion, different disorders and atypicalities seem to have different relentless preferences for explicitness and implicitness in terms of self-correction (Schegloff et al. 1977)

CONVERSATION ANALYSIS AND APHASIA

A variety of applied pragmatic approaches to aphasia exist. Here, the pragmatic tradition in the CA data-driven analysis of aphasic discourse will be described and discussed further. The value of the analytical CA approach is recognized widely. Hence, the pragmatic CA tradition will undergo a comparative analysis with a new analytical approach under construction—one formulated within an IL discursive framework. The IL-inspired framework borrows from the methodology of CA but ontologically differs markedly. This stance has interpretive implications for the analyst and for the outcome of the analysis. The IL-inspired analytical approach to the study of language disorders such as aphasic communication and autistic communication is a demonstrably different ontology. Thus, new insights into language disorders as social, individual, and societal phenomena may be gained by applying the IL perspective.

Traditionally, a participant's perspective is investigated through the observation of procedures followed by research interviews with the individuals about their experiences, including reflections, emotions, fears, and suggestions. This methodology is not impossible, but seems quite senseless when dealing with individuals with aphasia, whose major challenge, apart from other physiologically induced challenges, is the production of talk in dialogue, which is the basis of a research interview. Therefore, if research in the data-driven participatory experience of aphasia in everyday communication is to take place, a new analytical approach to uncover a participant's perspective needs to be developed. Researchers need to be able to grasp a participant's perspective and utilize that to be able, when necessary, to modify or improve procedures of aphasic discourse in health communication.

However, traditions in the study of aphasic discourse are strong. Multimodal studies have been carried out for the past 20 years with great success, and the insights gained are invaluable. Charles Goodwin (2000, 2003a) and Ray Wilkinson (2011, among others) have been major contributors in distributing knowledge on aphasic communication and in testing and training communication skills. Theirs is a data-driven multimodal approach, which investigates participatory meaning-making as a multiparty happening, where understandings and meanings are co-created with others. The multimodal approach is an applied CA approach, demonstrably based on the traditional methodology of CA. A multimodal applied CA approach to participatory meaning-making has long been the main key to access participatory understandings in interactions with individuals living with aphasia (Goodwin 2003a).

The methodology applied in many aphasic studies has its roots in traditional CA studies. As discussed in recent CA studies and literature, CA has evolved towards an augmented version of the traditional key CA principles. Newer CA studies investigate impairment and linguistic deficiency, aligning it with its studies in everyday conversations. This turn, ideologically, has a huge impact on "normalizing" all human interaction as simply communication by means of different styles by pointing to the fact that any communication could be categorized as atypical communication. Augmented CA, thus, is to be understood as an expansion of the area of interest of CA as much as an augmentation of the group of language users in question. Goodwin edited the key work on augmented CA, a multimodal CA approach in a study of "conversation and brain damage"—a book of that title (Goodwin 2003a).

The other major contributing scholar, Ray Wilkinson, has ventured into creating a credible frame for analysis using applied CA relevant for peers. The object studied once again is talk and coordination in conversations with persons with aphasia, their partners, and the therapists, doctors, and practitioners surrounding them (Wilkinson 2011, 2015). Furthermore, he has elaborated and tested intervention programs for recovery after aphasia (2011). In doing so, he has made major contributions to the restructuring of healthcare linguistic modules, hence improving care (Wilkinson 2011), and has contributed to methodologically demonstrating the usefulness of the standard CA forensic type of analysis. When the standard CA forensic type of analysis is applied to the study of communicational situations with interlocutors with aphasia and other brain injuries, it demonstrates that turn-taking rules apply even to conversations with people with very limited vocabularies. Goodwin demonstrated, in the case of Chill, how the availability of only three words ("yes," "no," and "du/and") was more than sufficient in order to be understood and to make oneself understandable (Goodwin 2003a). This study changed the view within interaction studies on impaired language and language disorders. From that time forward, multiple new study arenas opened up to researchers because Goodwin had enabled research to be undertaken on a whole new area of the lived life with brain damage, an area of study which previously had belonged to clinical studies and only investigated in isolated settings (Krummheuer 2015, p. 188).

Along with an augmented approach, more context is taken into consideration. As discussed by Goodwin, tsituational dialogues are part of a material coordination of other actions as well as involving other bodily expression than speech and gestures (Goodwin 2000; Krummheuer 2015). Goodwin's approach to the analysis of aphasic discourse from its early days regards it as fundamentally a question of cooperation:

> as an injury, aphasia does reside within the skull. However, as a form of life, a way of being and acting in the world in concert with others, its proper locus is a distributed multi-party-system. (Goodwin 1995, cited by Perkins 2003, p. 160)

Perkins (2003) points to the possibilities for rehabilitation and problem-solving tools to be developed from this stance, stating that CA provides unique and precise identification of "negotiated aphasia" (Perkins 2003, p. 160). By "negotiated aphasia," Perkins means aphasia dealt with sequentially in interaction in the applied CA tradition described by Goodwin (2003a), Wilkinson (2011).

A multimodal approach is not solely directed towards speech, as this differentiated focal area augments the observable units available for analysis (Goodwin 2000). The main tools in many CA analyses of aphasia and "negotiations of aphasia" in interactions are repair phenomena and repair negotiations (Perkins 2003). The organization of repair in aphasia is complex and differs from what Perkins labels "normal conversation." Also, the applied term of "understanding" as "positive evidence in the form of acknowledgement tokens or moving on to the next relevant contribution," or such phrasing as "understanding sufficient for current purposes" demonstrates well how CA describes social order as a distributed cognitive machinery in its overall terminology (Perkins 2003, p. 150). Hence, CA does not take an individual's experiential perspective into consideration, but remains a researcher-described interpretation of the individual's multiparty participatory meaning-making through their sequentially organized concert of a rule-governed social order, established with the tools from CA studies (Sacks et al. 1974; Schegloff 1968). Meaning-making, according to Goodwin and Wilkinson, is an intersubjectively shared matter, which is observed and grasped by observation and analyzed sequentially using a CA-based methodology and a CA-based ontology, which leans on the traditional next-turn proof-procedure (Sacks et al. 1974).

Turning to the idea of an IL analytical perspective, Duncker (2011) takes a new stance on "observable units" or "data" when she points to the fact that what really must matter to the integrationist is how the terms such as empirical, evidence, and data are construed (Duncker 2011, p. 533). What differs for the integrationist and the pure CA-analyst is exactly what is considered units of observance. When an IL perspective is sought to be applied, then the observer not only observes linguistic units or multimodal units, but also, and not least, the macroso-cial, biomechanical, and circumstantial factors of the communicational infrastructure. These shape the whole of the IL observation of phenom-ena and thus become the platform for the IL analysis, as discussed ear-lier in the case of distinguishing the object of observance as a matter of complementarity.

In aphasia studies, "non-ordinary" has been the descriptive categori-zation of the aphasic interlocutor's non-competence, which is defining aphasia. Perkins (2003) concludes on this basis, that the communicative non-ordinariness of the repair structure in aphasic interaction defines it as a difficult matter (Perkins 2003, p. 151). Yet, in this author's percep-tion, the category-problems in both autism research and aphasia research are ontological as well as philosophical. The bio-perspective produces a metaphorical terminology where mind and language are too closely linked. Simply put, sociality, the material setting, and circumstantial fac-tors are missing. This seems particularly to be the case in autism research as opposed to the counter-development in aphasia research, which has benefitted greatly from Goodwin's early ethnography studies, discussed in this chapter. However, as Perkins points out, making the organization of talk the problem also seems problematic in an IL perspective. This terminology presupposes language to have a preset normative structure, which the grounds of IL does not agree with.

The challenge of a dominant discursive bio-perspective is that it seems to be creating a danger zone of social stigmatization (Nielsen 2011, p. 599). In professional healthcare practice, the bio-perspective also plays a crucial role in the treatment of disorders other than autism. For instance, rehabilitating social interaction in institutional settings and in occupational and speech therapies draw on a bio-approach, as shown in the cases examined later in this book. By considering physical deficien-cies the causes of behavior, persons are no longer treated as persons but as clinical diagnoses without a well-founded understanding of the lived experience of the individual. This may lead to unintended social exclusion and violation of a person's right to personhood (Nielsen 2015; Sterponi 2004).

The obstacle of a dominant perspective, which discursively draws on the conceptualization of the existence of such thing as "atypical communication," is rather ontological to the integrationist. In an IL-view, whether considering autism or ABI, Nielsen (2011, 2015) points to explicit discourses which seem to generate emotional distress with the consequence of interactional discrepancy. This may point to problematic professional practices. This stated, Nielsen (2011, 2013, 2015), overlooks and fails to discuss the effects of having a disorder or disability on the individuals with impairment. Disorders are, by and large, physiologically rooted conditions which cause the deficiency in the first place.

NOTE

1. An updated version, the ICD-11 is expected in 2018.

REFERENCES

American Psychiatric Association. (2013). *Diagnostic and statistical manual of mental disorders DSM-5* (5th ed.). Arlington, VA: APA Publishing.

Antaki, C., & Wilkinson, R. (2013). Conversation analysis and the study of atypical populations. In J. Sidnell & T. Stivers (Eds.), *Handbook of conversation analysis* (pp. 533–550). Oxford: Blackwell Publishing.

Aphasiology. (1999). Special issue. *Conversation Analysis, 13*(4–5), 251–258.

Aphasiology. (2015). Special issue. *Conversation and Aphasia: Advances in Analysis and Intervention, 29*(3), 257–268.

Baron-Cohen, S., Leslie, A., & Frith, U. (1985). Does the autistic child have a "theory of mind"? *Cognition, 21*(19), 37–49.

Baron-Cohen, S. (1995). *Mindblindness: An essay on autism and theory of mind.* Cambridge, MA: MIT Press.

Björne, P. (2007). *A possible world.* PhD dissertation. Lund University, Cognitive Studies 134, Lund.

Brinkmann, S. (Ed.). (2010). *Det diagnosticerede liv.* Aarhus: Forlaget Klim.

Bøttcher, D., & Dammeyer, J. (2010). *Handicappsykologi: En grundbog om arbejdet med mennesker med funktionsnedsættelser.* København: Samfundslitteratur.

Duncker, D. (2011). On the empirical challenge to integrational studies in language. *Language Sciences, 33*(4), 533–543.

First, M., Frances, A., & Pincus, H. (2004). *DSM-IV-TR guide book.* Vancouver: American Psychiatric Publishing Inc.

Fleming, D. (1995). The search for an integrational account of language: Roy Harris and conversation analysis. *Language Sciences, 17*(1), 73–98.

Frith, U. (2003). *Autism: Explaining the enigma* (2nd ed.). Oxford: Blackwell Publishing.

Gergen, K. (2015). Toward a relational humanism. *The Journal of Humanistic Counseling, 54*(2), 149–165.

Goodwin, C. (2000). Action and embodiment within human interaction. *Journal of Pragmatics, 32*, 1489–1522.

Goodwin, C. (Ed.). (2003a). *Conversation and brain damage*. Oxford: Oxford University Press.

Goodwin, C. (2003b). Conversational frameworks for the accomplishment of meaning. In C. Goodwin (Ed.), *Conversation and brain damage* (pp. 90–116). Oxford: Oxford University Press.

Harris, R. (1996). *Signs, language and communication*. London: Routledge.

Harris, R. (1998). *Introduction to integrational linguistics*. Oxford: Pergamon.

Harris, R. (2004). Integrationism, language, mind and world. *Language Sciences, 26*(6), 727–739.

Harris, R. (2009). Integrating autism. *Integrationist notes and papers 2006–2008* (pp. 13–16). Gamlingay: Bright Pen.

Korkiakangas, T., Dindar, K., Laitila, A., & Kärnä, E. (2016). The Sally-Anne test: An interactional analysis of a dyadic assessment. *International Journal of Language and Communication Disorders, 51*(6), 685–702.

Krummheuer, A. (2015). Performing an action on cannot do: Participation, scaffolding and embodied interaction. *Journal of International Research in Communication Disorders, 6*(2), 187–210.

Leslie, A. (1987). Pretense and representation: The origins of "theory of mind". *Psychological Review, 94*(4), 412–426.

Leudar, I., & Costall, A. (Eds.). (2011). *Against theory of mind*. Basingstoke: Palgrave Macmillan.

Love, N. (2007). Are languages digital codes? *Language Sciences, 29*(5), 690–709.

McIlvenny, P. (1995). Seeing conversations: Analysing sign language talk. In P. ten Have & G. Psathas (Eds.), *Situated order: Studies in the social organisation of talk and embodied activities* (pp. 129–150). Washington, DC: University Press of America.

McIlvenny, P., & Raudaskoski, P. (1994). Sign language and deaf interaction: A preliminary study of sign talk in Northern Finland. In I. Ahlgren, B. Bergman, & M. Brennan (Eds.), *Perspectives in sign language usage* (pp. 269–291). Durham: The International Sign Linguistics Association.

Nielsen, C. (2011). Towards applied integrationism: Integrating autism in teaching and coaching sessions. *Language Sciences, 33*(4), 593–602.

Nielsen, C. (2013). *Integrating the mind: An analysis of the methaphorical terminology in autism research.* Guldbæk: Anvendt Ny Integrationel Lingvistik.

Nielsen, C. (2015). Senhjerneskade i et forståelsesperspektiv. S. Frimann, M. Sørensen, & H. Wentzer (Eds.), *Sammenhænge i sundhedskommunikation.* (pp. 247–281). Aalborg: Aalborg Universitetsforlag.

Pablé, A., & Hutton, C. (2015). *Signs, meaning and experience.* Berlin: De Gruyter Mouton.

Perkins, L. (2003). Negotiating repair in aphasic conversation: Interactional issues. In C. Goodwin (Ed.), *Conversation and brain damage* (pp. 147–162). Oxford: Oxford University Press.

Rae, J., & Ramey, M. (2015). Parents resources for facilitating the activities of children with autism at home. In J. N. Lester & M. O'Reilly (Eds.), *The Palgrave handbook of child mental health: Discourse and conversation studies* (pp. 459–479). Basingstoke: Palgrave Macmillan.

Raudaskoski, P. (2013). From understanding to participation: A relational approach to embodied practices. In T. Keisanen, E. Kärkkäinen, M. Rauniomaa, P. Siitonen, & M. Siromaa. (Eds.), *Multimodal discourses of participation, AfinLA yearbook* (Vol. 71, pp. 103–121). Jyväskylä: Suomen Soveltavan Kielitieteen Yhdistyks (AFinLA). ISSN 0781-0318.

Sacks, H., Schegloff, E., & Jefferson, G. (1974). A simplest systematics for the organization of turn-taking for conversation. *Language, 50*(4), 696–735.

Schegloff, E. A. (1968). Sequencing in conversational openings. *American Anthropologist, 70*(6), 1075–1095.

Schegloff, E., Sacks, H., & Jefferson, G. (1977). The preference for self-correction in the organization of repair in conversation. *Language, 53*(2), 361–382.

Simmons-Mackie, N., & Damico, J. (2008). Exposed and embedded corrections in aphasia therapy: Issues of voice and identity. *International Journal of Language and Communication Disorders, 43*(1), 5–17.

Sterponi, L. (2004). Construction of rules, accountability and moral identity by high-functioning children with autism. *Discourse Studies, 6*(2), 207–228.

Sterponi, L., & de Kirby, K. (2016). A multidimensional reappraisal of language in autism—Insights from a discourse analytic study. Special issue: Discourse and conversation analytic approaches to the study of autism spectrum disorders. *Journal of Autism Developmental Disorders, 46*, 394–405.

Tammet, D. (2006). *Born on a blue day: Inside the extraordinary mind of an autistic savant.* London: Hodder and Stoughton.

Toolan, M. (1996). *Total speech: An integrational linguistic approach to language.* Durham, NC: Duke University Press.

Wilkinson, R. (1999a). Introduction. *Aphasiology, 13*(4–5), 251–258.

Wilkinson, R. (1999b). Sequentiality as a problem and a resource for intersubjectivity in aphasic conversation: Analysis and implications for therapy. *Aphasiology, 13*(4–5), 327–343.

Wilkinson, R. (2011). Changing interactional behavior: Using conversation analysis in intervention programmes for aphasic conversation. In C. Antaki (Ed.), *Applied conversation analysis: Intervention and change in institutional talk* (pp. 32–53). Basingstoke: Palgrave Macmillan.

Wilkinson, R. (2015). Conversation and aphasia: Advances in analysis and intervention. *Aphasiology, 29*(3), 257–268.

Wilkinson, R., Lock, S., Bryan, K., & Sage, K. (2011). Interaction-focused intervention for acquired language disorders: Facilitating mutual adaptation in couples where one partner has aphasia. *International Journal of Speech-Language Pathology, 13*(1), 74–87.

World Health Organization. (2001). *The international classification of functioning, disability and health* ICF. Geneva: WHO.

World Health Organization. (2013). *How to use the ICF: A practical manual for using the international classification of functioning, disability and health.* Geneva: WHO.

World Health Organization. (2015). *International classification of health interventions* ICHI. Geneva: WHO.

World Health Organization. (2016). *International statistical classification of diseases and related health problems ICD-10* (10th ver., 2016 ed.). Geneva: WHO (Origin. 1992).

CHAPTER 4

Meaning—Towards a Person-Centered Approach

Abstract Traditionally, a cognitive model has been applied to assess clinical descriptions of output deficiencies in language disorders. On the other hand, the analytical basis of ethnomethodology and conversation analysis has contributed immensely to investigating shared understanding in social interaction, which has demonstrated the abledness of persons with language disorders refutably. This chapter suggests a new person-centered participant's perspective partially derived from ethnomethodology and conversation analysis. However, an integrational linguistic approach is missing in language and communication disorders. Approaching the topic of meaning-making practices in an integrational perspective, the author emphasizes the unique contextualization of lived language disorders with reference to a number of written accounts on lived disorders. Agreements and divergences between approaches are discussed.

Keywords Person-centeredness · Meaning-making · Contextualization
Agency

© The Author(s) 2018   45
C. M. B. Klemmensen, *Integrating the Participants' Perspective
in the Study of Language and Communication Disorders*,
https://doi.org/10.1007/978-3-319-78634-6_4

A New Person-Centered Meaning-Making

The interest in this book is directed towards questions about understanding the life-world, or *"Lebenswelt"* (Goodwin 2000, p. 1508), of persons with physiological and cognitive damages, and the affective challenges that everyday life offers. This introduction to meaning offers a theoretically founded preliminary establishment of a new participant perspective. The new participant perspective merges the participant perspective drawn from ethnomethodological traditions and a participant perspective drawn from the framework of IL. The uniquely person-centered approach of traditional language psychology lays the theoretical base of the author's discussion of meaning. The person-centered view of language and communication is central to Harris's semiotics (1996, 1998). Persons cannot be isolated from their language, and since persons are the ones, who undertake the enterprise of contextualizing, this invites a new analytical approach to the study of situated meaning-making. The new approach complementarily adds to current explorations of LCDs.

Person-Centeredness in Language and Communication Disorders

This introduction to meaning turns the spotlight towards the individual. As discussed in Chapter 3, an experiential awareness is advocated by the WHO's conceptual framework for the ICF model (WHO 2001, 2015). There is a call, both in professional and everyday discourse, to enhance understanding of the situation of the individual and their story (Charon 2001; Glintborg 2015; Grandin 2006, 2008; Leudar and Costall 2011). However, individuals with brain injury and autism have proved difficult for others to understand, and this condition is challenging for the individuals, their family, and lay-person peers in general (Björne 2007; Glintborg 2015; Nielsen 2011, 2013; Raudaskoski 2013).

Individuals with brain injury have limited abilities one way or another, challenging their participation in bodily and verbal communication as these abilities may be restricted or damaged. Further, this communicative prerequisite may effect interaction with professional practitioners and researchers in the field (Raudaskoski 2013). Accordingly, individuals with brain injuries may seem unaccountable as meaning-makers and, therefore, they are likely to be excluded from societal everyday life.

As mainstream theories and research on brain injury primarily focus on psychological and neurological issues of the brain itself, there is a lack of scientific knowledge on the social/communicative/interactional impact of impairment. Investigating dialogical intersubjectivity by enhancing the individual's experience of interaction and meaning-making has been suggested as a new perspective in health communication (for instance, Gillespie and Cornish 2010).

THE STATUS OF LANGUAGE IN LANGUAGE AND COMMUNICATION DISORDERS

Traditionally, a scientific understanding of LCDs inherently underscores approaching and studying "language." The measurable assessment of correct and incorrect performance has long been the order of the day in clinical tests. However, all performance may not be measurable or even captured by assessment tests. In continuation of the discussion in Chapter 2, language as the bearer of meaning has been given excessive attention (Harris 1998; Barad 2003, p. 802). The critique has been directed towards the cognitive language model, which EMCA studies have refuted. As discussed in the previous chapters, interaction studies have demonstrated discrepancies between clinical results of individuals with impairment and results acquired from social interaction studies (Dickerson et al. 2005; Leudar and Costall 2011).

MEANING-MAKING IN DIALOGICAL PRACTICES

Interaction is located in communication situations, which apply to the total entity of persons, sign production, and situation, following an integrational perspective (Harris 1998, p. 68). Like many dialogists, Harris considers meanings as the continuum of practices that humans go around doing (Márkova and Foppa 1990; Linell 2009). To start at the macro-level, generally, meaning-making is considered dialogical (Linell 1998). Dialogically, meaning-making is the activity that participants are engaged in when they are going around communicating in various situations. Moreover, this is validated by the analytical demonstration of persons often changing their opinions and understandings "as they go" (Linell 2009). The dialogical approach accounts for a dynamic strand in meaning, similar to the approach of IL.

SHARED MEANING-MAKING IN INTERACTION STUDIES

In all the phenomenologically oriented traditions after Garfinkel, the dynamics of understandings are investigated in various contexts (Goodwin 1979; Sacks 1984; Schegloff 1992; Heritage 1984). Accounts of dynamic meaning-making are investigated in interaction using recordings of the interactions. Traditionally, tape-recordings and transcripts of audible data served in the investigations. Today, video recordings and transcripts are used, which pose a challenge to transcription-techniques and accountability, due to the need to incorporate visual data, and advanced recording technology.

Within the EMCA tradition of CA, the analytical concepts of "taking turns" in dialogue and analytically operating a next-turn proof-procedure (Sacks et al. 1974, p. 729) are key concepts which commonly apply to the description and investigation of understandings. Understandings, or meaning-makings, are investigated as they are displayed explicitly while producing a turn, and demonstrated in a transcript of, for instance, a dialogue. Turn-taking and its organization is demonstrated by the analyst in the format of the transcript, while the next-turn proof-procedure is an analytical tool which validates an analyst's analysis of the displayed meaning-makings. As the notion "next-turn" implies, interaction is regarded as sequentially organized, which also accounts for the CA-idea that meaning in interaction may be repaired sequentially (Schegloff 1992). However, as discussed in Chapter 5, sequentiality may not explain all interaction phenomena in studies of LCDs. As discussed in Chapter 3, sequentiality, to some extent, has proved challenging in the study of aphasic communication, where the interaction is differently organized or, at least, sequences may be excessively delayed (Wilkinson 1999; Perkins 2003).

In interaction research, three main ways of describing understanding-in-interaction have dominated: first, in traditional EMCA, understandings of meaning are generally registered as minimal responses in the form of explicit interpretative linguistics signs; second, in elaborated versions of EMCA, such as in the work of John Heritage (1984), understandings of meaning may be described as they occur rather implicitly and only displayed in particles such as the token "oh," which analytically marks a supposed "change of state" in interaction; third, understandings of meaning may be described multimodally as they may be accounted for when displayed in intelligible gestures that serve as "semiotic resources" in interaction (Goodwin 2000, p. 1489).

Multimodal studies converted gestures to observable, semiotic units, giving the analyzable units status in line with the linguistic units in traditional linguistic analysis. Both analytical approaches create an ontological problem. Following an integrational critique, when linguistic or semiotic units are made analyzable, a new coding system arises (Fleming 1995). In consequence, CA does not correspond the idea that the entities, persons, and language exist only interdependently. The pragmatic aspects of aphasia research have been marked by an ethnographic interest for the past 50 years (Goodwin 1995). However, diagnostic criteria still strictly draw on clinical studies, which have been formulated from completely different backgrounds entangled in a traditional experimental research discourse, and a new analytical approach is still to unfold fully.

Methodological Issues Regarding Meaning-Making

At a general level, "sense-making" is approached in this book as a person's experienced understandings (Harris 1998; Conrad 2011; Nielsen 2015; Wiggins and Potter 2007). The investigation in this book is directed towards the methodological question of the extent to which a cross-disciplinary approach may help distinguish experienced communication as practiced by individuals from analysts' interpretations (Fleming 1995; Harris 2009; Sarangi 2007).

Currently, CA is the preferred approach in intervention studies (Rae and Ramey 2015; Wilkinson 2011, 2015). However, micro-analyses may not offer the overall picture. CA analyzes display and orientation that unfold during sequentially organized interaction. It cannot independently detect and analyze the processes this author wishes to describe regarding life-worlds (Abrams and Deniz 2015). For instance, we may not know from CA's abduction what a person understands beyond the social interaction they are engaged in (Roubillard 1996). The relevance of whether something is memorized correctly, for instance, will then depend on an augmented contextual configuration: which situations, persons, purposes, or connections are involved (Goodwin 2000, 2003; Harris 1998). However, we may, within CA's analytical concept of next-turn proof-procedure, describe organizational patterns of social interaction. Indeed, this may be a hypostasized way of uncovering enacted meaning in an integrational critique (Fleming 1995). However, a collaboration between CA and IL may work to some extent, as long as common orientation and divergences are discussed. For this reason, CA and IL are scrutinized and methodological and ontological divergences are identified.

A PERSON-CENTERED APPROACH TO MEANING

Meaning-Making in Language Psychology

Traditions in language psychology largely draw on EMCA (Nielsen 2012) and define communication as actual, situated practices, governed by individually determined structures of relevance (Hermann and Gregersen 1978; Gregersen 2004; Nielsen 2005, 2015), which configure how persons integrate meaning: their understanding of what they are trying to do (Goodwin 2000, pp. 1490–1492; Nielsen 2011).

Discursive psychology (DP) is considered to be a branch of contemporary language psychology (Nielsen 2012). It draws on EMCA and investigates social accomplishment and psychological display in everyday and institutional situations. Indeed, social order is in focus in DP, and therefore, this author considers DP to be a distributed social psychology rather than an individual psychology (Wiggins and Potter 2007; Jørgensen and Phillips 1999, pp. 105–120). However, a traditional language psychology defines interaction differently. It regards understanding and meaning-making as an individual enterprise carried out in situated and contextualized practices (Jespersen 1925; Mortensen 1953; Rasmussen 1980; Hermann and Folke Larsen 1973, 1974; Hermann and Gregersen 1978; Gregersen 2004; Rathje and Svenstrup 2004; Hermann et al. 2005). In addition, and as discussed by Nielsen (2015), language psychology is inclined more towards the integrational program of formulating a new general science of language. The integrational notion of contextualization and the concept of "relevance structure" from Danish language psychologists Jesper Hermann and Frans Gregersen (1978) are similarly unique: They single out a uniquely person-centered view on language and meaning grounded in a person's experiential history, rather than a socially oriented view popularized from DP and EMCA. This concept is closely linked to the practice theoretical concept of historical body, which is discussed in the following chapter.

Meanings Defined Integrationally

In an integrational view, meanings are defined as being attached to persons' experiences rather than to language. Crucially, Harris considers understandings first and foremost private and, in contrast to other interaction approaches, he points out that they may sometimes be implicit, which should be taken into account (Gillespie and Cornish 2010; Harris 2008; Ruus 1995). However, though meanings are regarded as private, the individual is subject to account for their social performance (Garfinkel 1967; Heritage 1984, p. 3). Therefore, the perception of unaccountable behavior produces problems in social interaction.

Methodologically, IL does not limit the analysis to the study of formal mechanisms in conversation in transcripts of various kinds, which Harris would consider scriptism (Fleming 1995, p. 73). Moreover, the notion of temporality is much wider in IL and not limited to the notion of a local sequentiality as in the case of CA. Ontologically, both are oriented towards uncovering lay-methods and a lay-rationality in social behavior. The divergence in ontology lies within the limitation of CA to the study of informal interaction, whereas IL covers premises about all language and communication. IL criticism of CA, for instance, has been directed at the normativity of the search for structures in interaction (Fleming 1995, p. 85). The procedural reproduction of structures in social interaction that IL advocates is a hypostasized entity which presupposes a system underneath the enactments: "a system unproblematically abstracted from particular events which it governs" (Fleming 1995, p. 85). As discussed in Chapter 2, as an alternative, Harris introduces three factors governing all communication: the biomechanical, the macrosocial, and the circumstantial factors. The problem of the system underneath leads to the main ontological divergence between CA and IL. The orientation towards situatedness within EMCA becomes a situatedness on the surface of structuring mechanisms (Fleming 1995, p. 88). Therefore, the CA fallacy in an IL perspective is that CA may end up studying the system at work rather than particular outcomes. After discussing a promising merging of CA and IL, Fleming (1995, p. 94) suggested a new panchronic analysis which would allow for contextualizing the present, the past, and the anticipated future in a meta-situated analysis. This would lead towards a new constructionism, which reaches beyond the limits of CA. Later, Fleming (1997) suggested such analysis would produce a close, detailed, empirical analysis of situated discursive action. Again, it may seem hard to distinguish CA from IL in Fleming's proposal. Therefore, this author will specify three things which may clarify the distinguishing features of CA and IL: first, meaning as it is applied in this book; second, how IL differs from CA; and third, pinpoint where the notion of meaning within IL diverges from the notion of meaning within CA.

Experiential Meaning

Historically, meanings and individual experience have been linked. Hans-Georg Gadamer, for instance, considered all understanding a response to something earlier understood (Gadamer 2004). In *The Principles of Psychology*, William James described habits and action patterns as interconnected to modes of understanding, since he considered meanings linked to self-perception and to the individual's acquisition of knowledge (James 1950, pp. 104–127; Nielsen and Hermann 2010). Contrastingly, Harold Garfinkel described meaning-making as socially shared in *Studies in Ethnomethodology* (1967), where he approached both visible and invisible conventions. In social interaction, Garfinkel studied how conventions were constantly challenged, broken, and repaired. In a line of experiments, he described situational rules.

Despite an ontological divergence between Gadamer, James, and Garfinkel regarding orientation towards the individual versus social meaning-making, the thoughts of these predecessors to IL all link two key notions more or less explicitly. First, the notion of experiential meaning (Pablé and Hutton 2015, p. 1). Second, the notion of situational meaning. In a similar fashion, Harris is concerned with articulating a science of language, which does not start with language but distinctly with the processual understandings of individuals communicating.

In *Integrationist Notes and Papers 2006–2008* (2009), Harris specifies that meanings are produced in the act of contextualization: meanings are values that are applied by persons as they are engaging in worldly matters. As stated, the consideration of situated meaning-making is a common orientation between EMCA and IL. Harris explicitly regards signs as the product of communication. In this view, the ongoing production of meanings is regarded as the very glue in interaction and intersubjectivity, which also applies to CA.

CONTEXTUALIZATION AND COTEMPORALITY

Harris offers two distinguishing theoretical concepts to apply in integrational language science, contextualization and cotemporality. These notions may lead to thoughts of EMCA; however, within IL the notions apply to approaching all language and communication, not solely to approaching informal social interaction as in the case of EMCA. The integrational concept of context is presented here for the first time in its extended version (for a summary, see Nielsen 2015). Contemporary summations of IL do not thoroughly deal with other aspects of the theoretical perspective than the currently revisited ontology of IL (for instance, Jones 2016; Love 2017; Cowley 2011; Linell 2015; Steffensen 2016, 2017).

Contextualization is a theoretical concept which describes "communicational context" (Harris 1998, p. 100). It also describes integrative activity, which communication is to be considered in an applied integrational perspective. Meaning that contextualization is to be regarded as an activity, a practice: the performing of individuals' flow of activities. Therefore, this author argues that IL is not to be understood as a mere ontology of "language" nor an intersubjective idealization (Jones 2016). IL is not strictly theoretical but takes a point of departure in descriptive practices of humans and is, thus, a concept which describes communicative activity and agency, and therefore it is applicable in empirical analyses (Fleming 1995). This is an overlooked feature. The distributed approach to language on the one hand aligns itself with dialogism but with claims of dealing with more embedded, enacted, extended and ecological aspects of cognition (4E) than, for instance, IL, innovating language science this way (Steffensen 2015, pp. 1–3). The 4E language view, on this ground, opposes itself to and discards a 3I language view, which considers language individual, internal and instrumental (Steffensen 2015, p. 3). Indeed, IL can be applied to describe action and practices, both individual and social, why this author discards the current distributed summation of IL.

Context as Agency

Meaning and context are inseparable to the integrationist. This view may be validated in many modern approaches to interaction and meaning-making. However, the integrational notion of contextualization is divergent and unique as it converts context to a matter of individual agency, as opposed to the traditional descriptions of context discussed in Chapter 2. As discussed by Linell (2015), persons, not the settings, are the ones who contextualize.

Humans contextualize as an ongoing activity in communication situations. Hence, meanings only exist as integrated by humans and their practices (Linell 2009). Contextualization is a descriptive concept, which embeds language and considers language as part of a larger activity process (Harris 1998, p. 98). As Linell (2015) points to, the distributed language theory does not contain an appropriated "dialogicality," since the focus on cognition as a dislocated concept merely separates humans from their minds and their activities.

Contextualization is a core concept in an applied integrational perspective. Hence, language cannot be studied in isolation but is always to be studied as a human feature and a process of contextualization. This point Harris demonstrates with the principle of cotemporality (Harris 1998, pp. 81–82):

> The chronological integration of language with events in our daily lives requires us to suppose that what is said is immediately relevant to the current situation, unless there is a reason to suppose otherwise. But this applies not only to what we say but also to everything we do. In other words, in this respect, there is a complete parity of status between linguistic acts and other acts. Linguistic acts do not have some special temporal status of their own, which somehow puts them outside the sequentiality of the rest of our existence [...] The way the principle of cotemporality impinges on semantics is as follows. It obliges the linguist to recognize that language does not provide us with miraculous guarantee of the stability of meaning(s) over time, or even from one moment to the next.

Cotemporality is demonstrated to depend on contextualization, thus contextualization conditions the principle of cotemporality. Harris elaborates on the concept of contextualization as he describes the concepts and the functions of the concepts of integration, chronology, and relevance. From here, he draws his concept of context as agency (contextualization): "Context is not some kind of neutral backdrop against which communication takes place" (Harris 2009, p. 71). Harris points to the argument that linguistic activity does not have a special status which separates it from the rest of our daily life activities. Linguistic activity is as contextualized as all the other activities we engage in that is integrated by ourselves (Harris 2009, p. 71):

> Context, for the integrationist, is always the product of contextualization, and each of us contextualizes in our own way, taking into account whatever factors seem to us to be relevant. The individual participants in any communication situation will each contextualize what happens differently, as a function of the integrational proficiency each exercises in that situation.

The concepts introduced above are to be understood as inseparable. The analytic consequence of semantic analysis is that "[…] determinacy is provided by the context of the activity" (Harris 1998, p. 101).

These concepts were introduced in Chapter 2; the analysis must be able to deal with semantic indeterminacy, contain the integration of understandings by actual individuals, and include the concepts contextualization and cotemporality. Together, these form the base of the threefold core of an applied integrational program of meaning. How to approach the individual's understandings analytically with this perspective in mind will be fully unfolded and explained further in the following chapters, which discuss integrationism as an analytical perspective. However, the path may be piloted by referring to the impact of the narrative medicine discourse. Due to the impact of this discourse, which advocates placing patient-centeredness at the heart of the analysis, currently, it makes sense to build and probe a theoretical argument to promote a new participant perspective within health communication, drawing on a person-centered view of language.

To Harris, an anecdotal narration is as reliable as a video recording, and this has nothing to do with cognitivist ideas. Simply, it is a matter of allowing persons to share understandings. Therefore, explicitness and implicitness in practices of understanding, whether displayed simultaneously or during recontextualization in narratives, are no different to the integrationist. Both display and contextualize, equally, persons' experiences of communication and consider how understanding and perception changes with time. Therefore, narratives such as literary cases on lived language disorders are interesting to study comparatively to analysts' findings as they, sometimes, do refute observable behaviors. Therefore, this author claims that the more "technical" the analysis, the less "humanly" it may treat the experiential nature of the interaction (Nielsen 2015).

An Alternative Theorizing on Language and Communication

IL and its potential analytical perspective are twofold. First, it is creating an outline for the possible application of an alternative theorizing on language and communication. Second, it is developing a potential methodology for analysis based on new basic assumptions regarding signs and meaning.

Structuralism's Heritage: Inherent Meaning in Language

As discussed in Chapter 2, in traditional linguistics, the interpretive content of scientific descriptions of sense-making have been based exclusively on the observation and description of visible and audible linguistic and extra-linguistic signs. Accordingly, this structuralism-based sign theory regards the content of signs as a mirror of historically structured systems of meaning ordered in "language." In other words, the structuralism-based assumption of language is that signs are inherent materialized reflections of a representational language system. In this view, the system itself is what generates the meanings negotiated culturally and historically and recorded in language. Consequently, meaning is presupposed to lead back to or to "represent" something: ideas, objects, phenomena, events, perceptions, or direct experiences. In a structuralist view, language users pick meanings from the representational preestablished historical body of language and meaning. However, questions about whose perception and experience it might be are nowhere addressed in structuralism. Crucially, the question of agency is central to the integrationist position on signs and meaning.

The Ascription of Content to the Sign

In structuralism, content (the signified) has the status of a reflection of something else, which is what ascribes content as inherent to language. Moreover, it objectivizes meaning, as structuralism assumes that the signification is a reflected phenomenon arbitrarily encapsulated in a sign. In this view, content is attached to language and not to actions. Signification is derived from its linguistic representation. This heritage from Saussure's theory of signs is based on the idea that meaning is assumed to be present in the very representation (the sign: the signifier and the signified).

First-Order and Second-Order Language

Recently, a renewed critique of structuralism has risen. Integrational linguists and advocates of the distributed language view share a common theoretical interest in changing the ontological status of language as an object of study. Together, they are changing the agenda of the way language is studied and discussed, at least in some areas of the language sciences (see, for instance, Pablé and Hutton 2015; Thibault 2011; Cowley 2011; Steffensen 2016; Pablé 2017).

A concept that integrational linguists and advocates of the distributed language view agree upon is the one that Nigel Love and Paul Thibault have taken up. They suggest distinguishing between two orders of language to explain the problem of structuralism's ontology. The two orders of language currently investigated within the language sciences they label "first-order" and "second-order" (Love 2007; Thibault 2011). First-order language covers the creative, informal, and often disorderly use of language between actual persons (Love 2007, 2017; Thibault 2011). CA may be said to study first-order language in the sense that negotiation of shared meaning is what is primarily investigated in dialogues. On the other hand, second-order language refers to the neat language described in the paragraphs above on structuralism and its heritage. Second-order language is what traditional linguists are studying systematically. Therefore, linguistic determinacy becomes an issue. The above distinction of the signifier from the signified is what categorizes the linguistic notion of language as a second-order phenomenon. From an IL perspective, second-order phenomena are by nature not reproducible of first-order experiences. First-order experiences unfold in time and, progressively emerge. Therefore, first-order experiences are largely driven by the suspense of linguistic indeterminacy (Pablé and Hutton 2015, pp. 28–29, 59; Orman 2017).

INTEGRATIONAL MEANING-MAKING

The notion of the second-order category is a way to express the basic axioms of an integrational semiology: an integrational position on signs and meaning. Signs do not exist as given items in a system of language. Therefore, signs and their meaning are considered the very result of the ongoing activity we call communication. Moreover, signification is not regarded as mirrored and reflected in a sign itself but considered "a function of the integrational proficiency which its identification and interpretation presuppose" (Harris 1996, p. 154). Content is meaning in the making, and signification exists only as part of somebody's communicative enterprise; signification is a direct experience of the perceivable meaningfulness of something to someone. It cannot preexist as a reflection of a meaning inherent in language, nor as a reflection of someone else's materially recorded experience. In an integrationist perspective, meaning encapsulated within a predetermined system such as language is merely a myth (Harris 1981). Still, it is categorized as a second-order phenomenon.

An Applied Integrational Linguistic Premise

Rather, integrationism is to be considered an account for why we often do not agree on something (Harris 2009, p. 71). An applied integrational agenda must include a broad definition of a communication situation, since it is the personal integration of an individual's own understandings which is the interactional premise. In CA, the interactional focus is different (e.g. Pomerantz and Fehr 1997). A scenario of understanding, or of interaction in isolation, cannot be the object studied within an applied integrational perspective (Fleming 1995, 1997). However, the object studied is how actual persons integrate their own understandings of what they are trying to do as the go about doing it. Therefore, an applied integrational perspective sheds light upon what persons are doing in and with their language. Hence, it is clarified by the very premise of an applied IL, that the object of study calls for interdisciplinarity. The study of actual persons and their integration of what they are trying to do as they go about doing it overlaps with the approach of practice studies (Nicolini 2012). This author points to the very premise of an applied IL in order to qualify its practice affordance. This is done in order to position it closer to practice studies with the purpose of considering it an ecological approach to the study of language and communication.

THE DISTRIBUTED LANGUAGE VIEW
AND INTEGRATIONAL LINGUISTICS

As mentioned above, an applied integrational perspective has little to do with the distributed language view and theory (Cowley 2011; Steffensen 2016). Since the early 2000s, several embodiment perspectives have been debated and discussed. In particular, notions of the concepts of "language" and "cognition" as phenomena distributed among more than one person (Cowley 2011; Linell 2013, 2015; Steffensen 2015, 2016). Other schools, including IL, have criticized the concepts of a distributed mind/cognition and a distributed language. Seemingly, to IL theorists, it is impossible to localize such a mind, cognition, or language (Harris 2004; Orman 2016). In contrast, the embodied perspective of IL is very easy to localize, since it is embodied in an individual person's body and mind. Summarizing, the uncommon ground between the distributed language view and IL: ontological similarities may be traceable. This way the anti-structuralism-ontology presented could be co-operated. However,

Steffensen (2016) deduces IL to be a mere criticism of twentieth-century general linguistics and fails to see the theoretical potential of qualifying IL as an applied science. Rather, he refers to integrationism as a critical voice to bring to bear when challenged by common beliefs of the language myth (see Harris 2004; Love 2004). The very core of this discussion leaves no doubt, however, about a categorical difference between the distributed mind, cognition and language views, and IL. Even the concept of distribution is claimed a "category mistake" by integrationists (Harris 2004; Orman 2016). This leads us to the diverged path. The premise of IL is founded in a general theory of language and communication, which build on the very persons communicating, something which is sharply underpinned. Moreover, this premise seems to be the main distinguishing feature and the "(un)common ground," to put it in Orman's words (2016), between the distributed view and the IL perspective. Discussing the role of will also causes these two paths to diverge where an integrational approach insists on an individual take but is willing to discuss the intentionality and autonomy of such a being, at least as a localizable one, for a start. In short, as Pablé and Hutton (2015) intensely underpin the embodied aspect of IL, "even if the self is not autonomous, it is nonetheless uniquely situated at the intersection of semiological processes" (Pablé and Hutton 2015, p. 5).

OPERATING ON THE GROUNDS OF AN INTEGRATIONAL LINGUISTIC PERSPECTIVE

Consequently, an IL perspective must work out a broad concept and a unique definition of "communication." As stated above, the persons communicating are at the center of this approach. Hence, "understanding" is not just a matter of interaction patterns but must also incorporate personal integration of one's own understandings. This person-centered premise is quite different from the interaction-centered focus in CA (Pomerantz and Fehr 1997). Since Harris states that the concept of "context" is not a "neutral backdrop against which communication takes place" (Harris 2009, p. 71), then, it must follow, that the object studied cannot be a scenario of understanding nor the interaction patterns in isolation, when approaching meaning-making integrationally. The object of study in an IL perspective is opposite by nature. It studies how actual persons integrate their own understandings of what they are trying to do as they go about doing it. Therefore, an analytical aspect of the IL perspective should approach and study more closely what actual persons are doing in and with their language.

Decompartmentalizing Linguistics

As demonstrated above, IL departs from both a compartmentalized, traditional general linguistics and from a structuralism-based, modern applied linguistics. These assume inherent systems of meaning in the traditional Saussurean sense. Consequently, the IL perspective is moving towards "a non-compartmentalized study of human interaction" (Pablé and Hutton 2015, p. 59). Epistemologically and ontologically, it suggests a radical sign theory and an alternative to traditional notions of "meaning as something inherent in signs." Finally, it informs the established tradition in modern applied linguistics with an important supplement.

Language Matters

Critics of the excessive focus on "language" itself are forced to venture into cross-disciplinary studies, which are broadening the object of study from "language" to, for instance, "agency," or "communication." For example, Karen Barad's agential realism (AR) focuses uniquely on agency (Barad 2003, 2007). Barad attributes agency to human and non-human agents (material objects), and their emergent flux practices, meaning matter's overall performativity. This way, Barad foregrounds non-human agents entangled trajectories, not persons (Barad 2007). Obviously, the biomechanical factors in language disorders may be approached and investigated this way, say in a clinical perspective. However, this author limits the interest to concern situated meaning.

As demonstrated above, the study may be broadened immensely when language is not the object studied, for example, when entities, persons, and language are regarded to exist only interdependently. In this view, the agential realist Barad and the IL approach agree. However, when discussing more closely the question of meaning and agency, it becomes clear that AR and an integrational approach diverge. Despite a shared interest in emergent practices and a preference for a common anti-fixed-code linguistic model, the presupposed localization of meanings and meaning-making differ greatly between AR (Barad 2003, 2007) and integrationism (Harris 1996, 1998). AR draws on performativity in human and non-human agents (stuff's performativity), whereas the integrational approach is concerned with the agency of human agents exclusively.

Towards a New Participant Perspective

Narrations of Language Disorders Included

In a new analytical perspective, persons with impairments are placed at the center of the analysis. This alternative conceptualization of a participant perspective is discussed by Nielsen (2011), drawing on Harris's semiotics. A similar conceptualization is that of Ivan Leudar and Alan Costall (2011), who draw on critiques of the dominant Theory of Mind discourse in autism research, discussed in Chapter 3. Overall, they align with a growing interest in considering the perspective of the individual through their narratives or an impaired perspective conceptualized in interaction analyses of individuals with disorders. Convincingly, a trend is traceable both inside and outside of academia. For instance, the volume of literature on the pragmatic understanding of others written by authors with autism has increased. As introduced by Nielsen (2011), drawing on the insights of Harris's analysis of Daniel Tammet's biography, *Born on a blue day* (2006), and her own commentary on Temple Grandin's biographies, *Thinking in Pictures: My Life with Autism* (2006) and *The Way I See it: A Personal Look at Autism and Asperger's* (2008), the idea gathers strength that the analyst approaches meaning-making in a participant perspective in the study of language disorders through native narratives, not only through surface-interaction analysis or clinical tests, which have been the dominant paradigm-strategies [like the argument of Leudar and Costall (2011)].

The above accounts serve as supplementary documents that demonstrate a real need for research attention (Clarke 2005). Furthermore, they portray the emotional side of living with impairments, which are themes that are excessively downscaled in traditional investigations of lived language disorders, apart from within the discourse of narrative medicine. Theoretically, they introduce a practice perspective, which helps augment the framework for the analysis of lived language disorders. The narrations of individuals with language disorders are useful for the purpose of triangulating and supplementing a strict interaction approach and a strict clinical approach to language disorders. Indeed, narrative accounts are challenging clinical psychology's one-faced descriptions of individuals with autism and brain injuries. For instance, going back to

Nielsen's discussion of Harris's examination of Daniel Tammet's narrative (Nielsen 2011), Harris (2009, pp. 13–16) points to characteristics of Tammet's story which shows that Tammet indeed experienced communication alternatively. His response to the teacher's questions were made, he just did not say them out aloud because he claimed not to feel this activity-engagement necessary. When Harris discusses this literary case, he explains that Tammet demonstrates explicitly that he did, in fact, understand the teacher's question linguistically, and that he responded a way relevant to his life-world. In sum, he did not fail to understand "language" nor to interact, which he did implicitly; however, he failed to behave in the socially expected manner. The unsaid expectation was that he would integrate by participating in the classroom practice, which is shared meaning in interaction, with the teacher and the other students in the classroom. Hereby, he oriented to an unaccountable interactional behavior, not an unaccountable understanding of language (Harris 2009; Nielsen 2011, p. 596). Similarly, Nielsen (2011) has discussed the biographies of the autistic researcher Temple Grandin, and anecdotes from her mentor experience with individuals with Asperger's.

Another distinct academic narration worth mentioning is the account of Albert Roubillard (1996). Because of the author's EMCA-proficiency, his account of being impaired himself concisely demonstrates the step by step, non-democratic, interactional order (Abrams and Deniz 2015) that his disability and impaired communication affords. Its social consequence results in a bitter life-world for him as an individual with impairment. Importantly, as discussed by Nielsen (2011, pp. 595–598), individuals with language impairment account for their individual meaning-making strategies.

The Beginning of Integrational Linguistic Analysis

Analyses carried out with an IL approach to the study of language and communication alter the status of observable units and the interpretation of their content. For instance, the study of dialogue dynamics in modern applied linguistics draws on presuppositions of orderliness and normativity in language use, and thus points to a traditional framework. The starting point for the development of an IL methodology is the integration of theories of IL into the workings of language and communication, and to consider and describe the mythical assumption-based framework of structuralism, which still dominates basic beliefs about the signification of displays in EMCA (Harris 1996, 1998; Toolan 1996; Fleming 1995; Love 2007; Pablé and Hutton 2015).

Research Questions

This research framework is limited to investigating the consequences of brain injury in interaction with health professionals and peers in everyday life. Therefore, the research questions are the following:

- What are the consequences of LCDs, and ABI in everyday practices?
- How can communications be described as participation abilities, drawing on a joint framework: contextualization from IL and the conventions of EMCA?
- How can communications be described through an empirical study on communication difficulties, combining the approach of IL and EMCA?
- Can the theoretical-analytical framework be organized and applied so that both practitioners and peers can validly use the model to analyze situated understanding?

The questions are investigated through a cross-disciplinary approach, which is outlined in the overlap of ethnography, anthropological medicine, communication research, and language psychology. It is important to repeat that the English words "how-abled" (Raudaskoski 2013) versus the term "disabled" frame the approach for this investigation of linguistic impairment and ABI, the resources for mutual understanding, and inclusion and exclusion practices. In short, a person-centered view on communication-as-practice is drawn within an already established field with the purpose of developing a methodological resource available for further empirical and theoretical investigation.

Essentially, a new approach with a clearer statement of the relationship between language, persons, and meaning is needed in order to properly link persons dealing with impairments and their communicational practices versus language-idea-based relations between displays of linguistic and extra-linguistic signs, whether produced in cognitive tests, everyday interaction, or in rehabilitation and occupational therapy. Quite possibly, more attention towards the individual in health-related matters may improve society's understanding of LCDs. This is of great social importance to individuals living with diagnoses such as brain injury, autism, and language disorders in general, since these groups of individuals often are challenged in understanding. A person-centered approach may help facilitate understanding and, accordingly, increase inclusion and improve treatment.

CONCLUSION

The object of study in IL is limited to the investigation of the relationship between the individual's meaning-making practices. Certainly, materials and culture matter to the integrationist. However, the central concern to IL is the radical indeterminacy of language, which is raised by individuals involved in situated meaning-making. Therefore, individuals' meaning-making is regarded the key analytical concern. This key concern links IL closely to narrative medicine in health-related studies, such as the study of language disorders. More generally, IL is concerned with mythological beliefs about language as an object of study, which is inherent to the sciences of language (Harris 1981, 1996, 1998, 2009).

Importantly, the notion of "integrational" grounds meaning-making in someone's experience as a person rather than formally in social interaction in material settings. Therefore, meaning-making practices, in an integrational sense, are not simply meaning-making-practices. Rather, the individual activity of meaning-making is labeled "contextualization," since this refers to an individual agency. However, as demonstrated in this chapter, there are strong theoretical alliances between EMCA, DP, the distributed language view, AR, and IL. Persuasively, the ontology of IL and traditional language psychology position these closer to one another than the other approaches, when regarding meaning.

REFERENCES

Abrams, T., & Deniz, G. (2015). Accounting for disability in the phenomenological life-world. *Journal of Existential and Phenomenological Theory and Culture, 10*, 1–23.

Barad, K. (2003). Posthumanist performativity: Toward an understanding of how matter comes to matter. *Signs: Journal of Women in Culture and Society, 28*(3), 801–831.

Barad, K. (2007). *Meeting the universe halfway: Quantum physics and the entanglement of matter and meaning.* Durham, NC: Duke University Press.

Björne, P. (2007). A possible world. PhD dissertation, Lund University, Cognitive Studies 134, Lund.

Charon, R. (2001). Narrative medicine: A model for empathy, reflection, profession, and trust. *Journal of American Medical Association, 286*(15), 1897–1902.

Clarke, A. (2005). *Situational analysis: Grounded theory after the postmodern turn.* Thousand Oaks, CA: Sage.

Conrad, C. (2011). Forståelseshandlingen: En empirisk afprøvet teori om narrativ forståelse som situeret betydning i dannelse. PhD dissertation, Københavns Universitet, København.

Cowley, S. (Ed.). (2011). *Distributed language.* Amsterdam: John Benjamins.

Dickerson, P., Rae, J., Stribling, P., Dautenhahn, K., & Werry, I. (2005). Autistic children's co-ordination of gaze and talk: Re-examining the 'asocial' autist. In K. Richards & P. Seedhouse (Eds.), *Applying conversation analysis* (pp. 19–37). Basingstoke: Palgrave Macmillan.

Fleming, D. (1995). The search for an integrational account of language: Roy Harris and conversation analysis. *Language Sciences, 17*(1), 73–98.

Fleming, D. (1997). Is ethnomethodological conversation analysis an "integrational" account of language? In G. Wolf & N. Love (Eds.), *Linguistics inside out* (pp. 182–207). Amsterdam: John Benjamins.

Gadamer, H. (2004). *Sandhed og metode* (A. Jørgensen, Trans.). Aarhus: Systime (Origin. 1960).

Garfinkel, H. (1967). Studies of the routine grounds of everyday activities. In G. Psathas (Ed.), *Studies in ethnomethodology* (pp. 35–75). Cambridge: Polity Press.

Gillespie, A., & Cornish, F. (2010). Intersubjectivity: Towards a dialogical analysis. *Journal for the Theory of Social Behaviour, 40*(1), 19–46.

Glintborg, C. (2015). Disabled and not normal: Identity construction after an acquired brain injury. *Narrative Inquiry, 25*(1), 1–21.

Goodwin, C. (1979). The interactive construction of a sentence in natural conversation. In G. Psathas (Ed.), *Studies in ethnomethodology* (pp. 97–121). New York: Irvington Publishers.

Goodwin, C. (1995). Co-constructing meaning in conversation with an aphasic man. *Research on Language and Social Interaction, 28*(3), 233–260.

Goodwin, C. (2000). Action and embodiment within human interaction. *Journal of Pragmatics, 32*, 1489–1522.

Goodwin, C. (Ed.). (2003). *Conversation and brain damage.* Oxford: Oxford University Press.

Grandin, T. (2006). *Thinking in pictures: My life with autism* (2nd ed.). New York: Vintage Books.

Grandin, T. (2008). *The way I see it: A personal look at autism and Asperger's.* Arlington: Future Horizons.

Gregersen, F. (2004). Fem eller seks slags forståelse. In M. Rathje & L. Svenstrup (Eds.), *Sprogpsykologi - udvalgte kerneemner* (pp. 67–77). København: Museum Tusculanum.

Harris, R. (1981). *The language myth.* London: Duckworth.

Harris, R. (1996). *Signs, language and communication.* London: Routledge.

Harris, R. (1998). *Introduction to integrational linguistics.* Oxford: Pergamon.

Harris, R. (2004). Integrationism, language, mind and world. *Language Sciences, 26*(6), 727–739.

Harris, R. (2008). *Mindboggling - preliminaries to a science of the mind*. Luton: Pantaneto Press.

Harris, R. (2009). *Integrationist notes and papers 2006–2008*. Gamlingay: Bright Pen.

Heritage, J. (1984). *Garfinkel and ethnomethodology*. Oxford: Basil Blackwell.

Hermann, J., & Folke Larsen, S. (1973). Sprogforståelse og erfaringsbaggrund. *Dansk Psykolog Nyt, 20*, 371–375.

Hermann, J., & Folke Larsen, S. (1974). "Forståelse" som sprogpsykologisk begreb. *SAML, 1*, 71–81.

Hermann, J., & Gregersen, F. (1978). *Gennem sproget; om undersøgelse af sprogbrug i samfundet*. Copenhagen: Gyldendal.

Hermann, J., Siiner, M., & Nielsen, C. (Eds.). (2005). *På sporet af sprogpsykologi - 12 artikler om sproglighedens psykologi*. København: Frydenlund.

James, W. (1950). *The principles of psychology* (Vols. 1–2). Cambridge, MA: Harvard University Press (Origin. 1890).

Jespersen, O. (1925). *Menneskehed, nasjon og individ i sproget*. Oslo: Aschehoug.

Jones, P. E. (2016). "Coordination" (Herbert H Clark), "integration" (Roy Harris) and the foundations of communication theory: Common ground or competing visions? *Language Sciences, 53*, 31–43.

Jørgensen, M., & Phillips, L. (1999). *Diskursanalyse som teori og metode* (pp. 105–120). Roskilde: Roskilde Universitetsforlag, Samfundslitteratur.

Leudar, I., & Costall, A. (Eds.). (2011). *Against theory of mind*. Basingstoke: Palgrave Macmillan.

Linell, P. (1998). *Approaching dialogue*. Amsterdam: John Benjamins.

Linell, P. (2009). *Rethinking language, mind, and world dialogically*. Charlotte, NC: Information Age Publishing.

Linell, P. (2013). Distributed language theory, with or without dialogue. *Language Sciences, 40*, 168–173.

Linell, P. (2015). Dialogism and the distributed language approach: A rejoinder to Steffensen. *Language Sciences, 50*, 120–126.

Love, N. (2004). Cognition and the language myth. Distributed cognition and integrational linguistics. *Language Sciences, 26*(6), 525–544.

Love, N. (2007). Are languages digital codes? *Language Sciences, 29*(5), 690–709.

Love, N. (2017). On languaging and languages. *Language Sciences, 61*, 1–35.

Márkova, I., & Foppa, K. (1990). *The dynamics of dialogue*. London: Harvester Wheatsheaf.

Mortensen, A. (1953). *Perception og sprog: Et filosofisk essay*. København: Akademisk forlag.

Nicolini, D. (2012). *Practice theory, work, and organization: An introduction*. Oxford: Oxford University Press.

Nielsen, C. (2005). Perception som forståelsens grundlag. In J. Hermann, C. Nielsen, & M. Siiner (Eds.), *På sporet af sprogpsykologi - 12 artikler om sproglighedens psykologi* (pp. 15–26). København: Frydenlund.

Nielsen, C. (2011). Towards applied integrationism: Integrating autism in teaching and coaching sessions. *Language Sciences, 33*(4), 593–602.

Nielsen, S. (2012). *Sprogpsykologi: Det teoretiske grundlag*. København: Samfundslitteratur.

Nielsen, C. (2013). *Integrating the mind: An analysis of the methaphorical terminology in autism research*. Guldbæk: Anvendt Ny Integrationel Lingvistik.

Nielsen, C. (2015). Senhjerneskade i et forståelsesperspektiv. In S. Frimann, M. Sørensen, & H. Wentzer (Eds.), *Sammenhænge i sundhedskommunikation* (pp. 247–281). Aalborg: Aalborg Universitetsforlag.

Nielsen, C., & Hermann, J. (2010). Tankestrømmens usynlige tråde. *Spindet, 10*(1), 50–52.

Orman, J. (2016). Distributing mind, cognition and language: Exploring the (un)common ground with integrational linguistics. *Language and Cognition, 8*(1), 142–166.

Orman, J. (2017). Indeterminacy in sociolinguistics and integrationist theory. In A. Pablé (Ed.), *Critical humanist perspectives: The integrational turn in philosophy of language and communication* (pp. 96–113). London: Routledge.

Pablé, A., & Hutton, C. (2015). *Signs, meaning and experience*. Berlin: De Gruyter Mouton.

Pablé, A. (Ed.). (2017). *Critical humanist perspectives: The integrational turn in philosophy of language*. London: Routledge.

Perkins, L. (2003). Negotiating repair in aphasic conversation: Interactional issues. In C. Goodwin (Ed.), *Conversation and brain damage* (pp. 147–162). Oxford: Oxford University Press.

Pomerantz, A., & Fehr, J. B. (1997). Conversation analysis: An approach to the study of social action as sense making practices. In T. van Dijk (Ed.), *Discourse as social interaction* (pp. 64–91). London: Sage.

Rae, J., & Ramey, M. (2015). Parents resources for facilitating the activities of children with autism at home. In J. N. Lester & M. O'Reilly (Eds.), *The Palgrave handbook of child mental health: Discourse and conversation studies* (pp. 459–479). Basingstoke: Palgrave Macmillan.

Rasmussen, E. (1980). *Om emners fremtræden og om forståelse som særligt emne: Undersøgelser over erkendelsen*. Københavns Universitet: Psykologisk laboratorium.

Rathje, M., & Svenstrup, L. (Eds.). (2004). *Sprogpsykologi - udvalgte kerneemner*. København: Museum Tusculanum.

Raudaskoski, P. (2013). From understanding to participation: A relational approach to embodied practices. In T. Keisanen, E. Kärkkäinen, M. Rauniomaa, P. Siitonen, & M. Siromaa. (Eds.), *Multimodal discourses of participation, AfinLA yearbook* (Vol. 71, pp. 103–121). Jyväskylä: Suomen Soveltavan Kielitieteen Yhdistyks (AFinLA).

Roubillard, A. B. (1996). Anger in-the-social-order. *Body and Society, 2*(1), 17–30.

Ruus, H. (1995). *Danske kerneord* (Vol. 1, pp. 3–18). København: Museum Tusculanum.

Sacks, H. (1984). On doing "being ordinary". In J. Atkinson & J. Heritage (Eds.), *Structures of social action: Studies in conversation analysis* (pp. 413–429). Cambridge: Cambridge University Press.

Sacks, H., Schegloff, E., & Jefferson, G. (1974). A simplest systematics for the organization of turn-taking for conversation. *Language, 50*(4), 696–735.

Sarangi, S. (2007). The anatomy of interpretation: Coming to terms with the analyst's paradox in professional discourse studies. *Text and Talk, 27*(5/6), 567–584.

Schegloff, E. (1992). Repair after next turn: The last structurally provided defense of intersubjectivity in conversation. *American Journal of Sociology, 97*(5), 1295–1345.

Steffensen, S. (2015). Distributed language and dialogism: Notes on non-locality, sense-making and interactivity. *Language Sciences, 50*, 105–119.

Steffensen, S. (2016). Sprogvidenskabens kognitive spørgsmål: En introduktion til den distribuerede sprogtilgang. *Nydanske Sprogstudier, 50*, 13–54.

Tammet, D. (2006). *Born on a blue day: Inside the extraordinary mind of an autistic savant*. London: Hodder and Stoughton.

Thibault, P. (2011). First-order languaging dynamics and second-order language: The distributed language view. *Ecological Psychology, 23*(3), 210–245.

Toolan, M. (1996). *Total speech: An integrational linguistic approach to language*. Durham, NC: Duke University Press.

Wiggins, S., & Potter, J. (2007). Discursive psychology. In C. Willig & W. Stainton-Rogers (Eds.), *The Sage handbook of qualitative research in psychology* (pp. 73–90). London: Sage.

Wilkinson, R. (1999). Sequentiality as a problem and a resource for intersubjectivity in aphasic conversation: Analysis and implications for therapy. *Aphasiology, 13*(4–5), 327–343.

Wilkinson, R. (2015). Conversation and aphasia: Advances in analysis and intervention. *Aphasiology, 29*(3), 257–268.

Wilkinson, R., Lock, S., Bryan, K., & Sage, K. (2011). Interaction-focused intervention for acquired language disorders: Facilitating mutual adaptation in couples where one partner has Aphasia. *International Journal of Speech-Language Pathology, 13*(1), 74–87.

World Health Organization (2001). *The International classification of functioning, disability and health ICF*. Geneva: WHO.

World Health Organization (2015). *International classification of health interventions ICHI*. Geneva: WHO.

CHAPTER 5

Introduction to the Preliminary Framework of a New Analytical Perspective

Abstract Approaches to language and communication disorders may substitute the notion of "language" with the analytical decoding of, for instance, talk, semiotic gesture, and emotional display. In this chapter, a non-telementational framework is presented as a new framework for approaching language and communication disorders. Tools inspired from practice theory, and concepts from integrational linguistics and ethnomethodology and conversation analysis are introduced in this joint framework. However, within integrational linguistics the notion of language (Harris 1981), linguistic models of language activity (Harris in Signs, language and communication, Routledge, London, 1996, Harris in Introduction to integrational linguistics, Pergamon, Oxford, 1998; Love in Lang Sci 61:1–35, 2017; Orman in Critical humanist perspectives: The integrational turn in philosophyof language and communication, Routledge, London, 2017), and data analysis (Duncker in Lang Sci 33:533–543, 2011; Fleming in Lang Sci 17:73–98, 1995, Fleming in Linguistics inside out, John Benjamins, Amsterdam, pp. 182–207, 1997; Toolan in Total speech: An integrational linguistic approach to language, Duke University Press, Durham, NC, 1996) are considered ontologically troublesome (second-order categories). Therefore, similarities and divergences between traditional models and the joined approaches are discussed by downgrading and discarding orthodox positioning.

© The Author(s) 2018
C. M. B. Klemmensen, *Integrating the Participants' Perspective
in the Study of Language and Communication Disorders*,
https://doi.org/10.1007/978-3-319-78634-6_5

Keywords Diffraction · Applied integrationism · Ethnomethodology and conversation analysis · Practice theory · Harmonization

THE CREATION OF AN APPROACH

This chapter joins several ends of this work with a threefold purpose. First, existing perspectives on language and communication disorders (LCDs) are introduced to attend quality of life (QOL)-related questions. As it will be discussed, individual perception is enhanced in QOL, which is highly relevant to the ambition of this book. Second, a focus on practices is enhanced as it replaces language in this new analytical perspective. Third, the participant perspective in ethnomethodology and conversation analysis program (EMCA) is elaborated with scrutiny to prepare its merging into a new participant's perspective. This methodology of giving attention to the differences of existing and divergent perspectives is labeled diffraction by Karen Barad (2007, p. 72). Diffraction is conceptualized from a physical phenomenon in the natural sciences but it is applied figuratively when referred to in practice studies.

Existing Analytical Approaches to Language and Communication Disorders

Multiple perspectives exist on LCDs. Current international approaches to the study of LCDs include three main approaches. Carol Legg and Claire Penn have listed them (2013, p. 18):

- The interactional approach (drawing on sociolinguistic tradition and social interaction studies discussed in Chapter 3)
- The insider approach (drawing on subjective, personal illness experiences and biographies, discussed in Chapter 4)
- The QOL approach (drawing on studies in real-life consequences of functional disorders and gains in rehabilitation processes aligned with the WHO frame, discussed in Chapters 3 and 4, and this chapter).

A shift from the social to the individual, and the development towards a societal framework approach to LCDs can be traced in the above. Most recent, the QOL approach draws on a multifaceted paradigm of disability, ability, and QOL, which includes contextual nuances. The WHO definition of QOL is grounded in the individual's perception of opportunities in life (WHO 1995, p. 164). This interprets in *disability studies* as "maximizing opportunities to participate fully in social, cultural, and economic life" (Warner and Manderson 2013, p. 1). This broad concept of QOL downgrades clinical facts and instrumentation to capture subjective assessment. Instead, it foregrounds a functional view which differentiates abledness, as described in Chapter 3. Importantly, QOL seemingly makes ethics, social justice and equity relevant topics, since the rights of people to enhance their capabilities is highlighted, as well as a demand for assessing the resources available to enhance these capabilities. In line with this view, social justice and the individual's access to resources also becomes a highly relevant topic.

This development is illustrated, for instance, in a QOL study conducted by Legg and Penn (2013). They followed impaired South Africans in a context study in particularly low-income areas. South Africa is highlighted as the country in the world with the highest number of strokes per year, as well as being described as a special case due to its unique sociocultural history. Their main findings are that uncertainty, vulnerability, and isolation characterize the lives of the impaired individuals and, therefore, their low life-quality measurement. Interestingly, similar notions of uncertainty, vulnerability, and social isolation are central in the findings of Chalotte Glintborg (2015, 2018), who has studied the psychosocial consequences individuals' lives post-stroke in a Danish context. The organization of health and social care in the case of Denmark is starkly different from the case of South Africa. Denmark is well-known for its welfare society and for high tax rates when compared to most other countries. Furthermore, it is known for its citizens' excellent access to health and social care and for its patient-safety policies. However, surprisingly, individuals with impairment in Denmark indicate similar low QOL as do the South Africans. In both these studies, individuals' QOL with lived LCDs are reported as low, regardless of access to care services, differentiated national socioeconomic status, and the rehabilitation provided. In sum, access to and accessing of health and social care are quite different, since programs and services may be available, but barriers to access (both formal and informal) and the need for individuals and families to organize care across sectors can impede the use of such services. Likewise, notions of loneliness and feelings of "not being normal" are retrieved as dominant in the Danish study (Glintborg 2015), similar to the South African study. Interestingly, the ideal ethical discourse from the International Classification of Functioning, Disability and Health (ICF) model is reflected in the recommendations for change retrieved from the real-world, pragmatic discourse studies.

An international study points to an overall need to improve the QOL of individuals with impairment through attention to psychosocial needs (Wallace et al. 2016). It calls for a family-centered approach to rehabilitation that will allow individuals to state personal needs in accordance with the ICF. This indicates a paradigmatic shift from the focus on clinical facts as measurements of QOL to a more nuanced focus on the individual and individual's rights (Wallace et al. 2016). This book further supports the call for enhancing a QOL focus in LCDs.

Language Disorders as Social Individuals' Lived Practices

As stated earlier, this book's focus is practice-based, and "lived disorders" refers to activities evolving around social, everyday lives of individuals with LCDs. This approach links to the QOL macro-framing, where social opportunities, participation, finding meaning in, and enjoyment of social and cultural activities are evaluated. The rights of people with impairments are relevant as they form part of the assessment of everyday participation capabilities (Nielsen 2015). The QOL approach is, therefore, to be considered a macro-framing of this book's approach.

A Practice Approach to Studying Language Disorders

Nexus Analysis as Action Tracer

Since this book revolves around practices, it is not interested in the micro-sequential organization of linguistic impairment; therefore, this analysis needs to be broadened. To capture practices such as routines and individual habits in material settings, larger frames are needed for the data analysis. The ethnographic approach nexus analysis (NA) (Scollon and Scollon 2004, 2007), which is derived from Mediated discourse analysis (MDA) (Scollon 2001), is concerned with uncovering the intersection of actions: the nexus of practice. The NA analyst applies a material-discursive approach, and can investigate situations in macro-frames as s/he is tracing the development of situational ecologies over time and through spaces. Change and emergent properties are converted to descriptive units and, this way, made observable and traceable to the analyst. In Scollon and Scollon's *Practical Fieldguide* (2004, pp. 152–178), tools are presented which guide the query of the analyst throughout the course of investigating and localizing the nexus of practice that s/he follows. NA provides the analyst with framing tools to create data that reflects how individual actors behave in social settings, through social affairs, and produce various outcomes with real consequences in situations, not just interactional divergence (Larsen and Raudaskoski 2016).

This book joins three different schools into a new analytical approach: practice theory (PT), integrational linguistics (IL), and EMCA. Together, these form a new approach, a person-centered praxeology that aims at focusing on consequences of social action rather than on new theorizing on the linguistic part of LCDs. The first part of this chapter and the first part of the following chapter are dedicated to discussing the PT backbone of this person-centered praxeology.

Understanding Practices: Practice Theory and Praxeology

Continuously, the notion praxeology covers the overall science and investigation of human action, whereas PT, in short, specifically covers praxeology as approach in a socially oriented version. Andreas Reckwitz (2002) has contributed to the formulation of a theory of social practices and configurations of the social. Apart from Ron Scollon and Suzie Scollon, other PT figures important to this approach include Theodore Schatzki, Johannes Angermüller, François Cooren, Adele Clarke, and last but not least, Davide Nicolini.

According to Nicolini, an eclectic strategy in PT analysis is common ground (Nicolini 2012). With this view, it makes little sense to search for one overall explanation of what PT is. Rather, PT approaches are a range of approaches whose main interest are to target the investigation of joint activities: the social and the workings of the social. Nexus analysis is one among several of such approaches. Nicolini (2012, p. 214) underlines that a unified approach within PT is non-existent. An overview of PT and its distinct features is bound to be confusing; however, main points are redundant in PT (Nicolini 2012, p. 217):

- Accomplishments are regarded as social by nature, also when attributed to individuals.
- Practices are considered mutually connected and constitutive of nexus, texture, field, and network.
- Intelligibility is a key.
- Epistemic objects uncovered account for practices.

In addition, PT adds something further than the focus on social structure found in EMCA. In contrast to EMCA, PT goes beyond "investigating practice 'as it happens'" (Nicolini 2012, p. 215). Moreover, the investigation of practice is linked to the concept "reality reconfiguration" in the sense that its objective is to thicken description and analysis and shed light on things that matter (Nicolini 2012, p. 217). The idea is to apply PT to "slice the social world." This data is available as practices are being re-presented in texts, by mapping of the world, or by linguistic conceptualization, simply, by applying a graphical technique which can show the interconnection of variables (Nicolini 2012, p. 218). This mapping may serve as a tool for investigating QOL-related aspects of LCDs and other quality-related assessments.

Traceability of Practices Across Temporal and Spatial Frames

Nicolini (2012) offers two main methodological "movements" to construct time and space-differentiation to localize the nexus of practice: "zooming in" and "zooming out."

Social accomplishments may be studied on a micro-level with the movement of zooming in, while the recognition of interrelated links across space and time are studied "sideways" with the movement of zooming out (Nicolini 2012, p. 219):

> zooming in on the accomplishments of practice; zooming out to discern their relationships in space and time; and using the above devices to produce diffracting machinations that enrich our understanding through thick textual renditions of mundane practices.

The mapping of trajectories, that is, the events and their recognizable features that emerge from the attention given them, demonstrate the location of a nexus of practice. Practices are not discourses but discursive, as they are presumed to exist only when enacted and re-enacted. In short, practices are "social and material doings" (Nicolini 2012, p. 221).

The Foundation of a Person-Centered Praxeology

The main purpose for diffracting approaches into a cross-disciplinary approach is to achieve a closer and a wider understanding (by zooming in and out) of how social practices in interaction may be studied in relation to inclusion and exclusion. The outset for establishing a person-centered praxeology is to study a participants' perspective in practices as they continuously unfold. The integrational concepts introduced in Chapter 2 (the biomechanical, the macrosocial, and the circumstantial factors) are applied to describe the history of a person's interactional behavior. The concept of historical body in NA and the IL-derived notion of the history of a person's interactional behavior are common ground. However, they differ analytically in the sense that NA considers social interaction a scenario, whereas IL considers an individual point of view. Apart from this distinct feature, they cover the same concept of human action.

Trouble sources in intervention and rehabilitation practices can be approached differently through the combined application of PT, IL, and EMCA. The main purpose of this data-driven approach is to establish a basis for the investigation of LCDs in practice. A by-product of engaging a combined IL and EMCA perspective in practice investigations is a further exploration of the theoretical differences and overlaps of the approaches that add new, original contribution to the theoretical corpora of both IL and EMCA. Fundamentally, understanding is regarded as an action underpinning the understandings of participants as they are producing them in discursive practice (Harris 1998; Conrad 2011; Wiggins and Potter 2007).

FROM A PRAGMATIC TO A SOCIETAL APPROACH TO LANGUAGE DISORDERS

A variety of applied pragmatic approaches to LCDs exist already, such as the widely recognized tradition of CA. As discussed in Chapter 4, a comparative analysis of CA and IL demonstrates both strong similarities and divergences. This discussion is continued as the new analytical approach is unfolding.

Discursive psychology (DP) is a program complementary to CA for investigating discursive practices. It draws extensively on the methods and findings of CA, hence the link between DP and CA is inseparable. The above-mentioned introduction to DP emphasizes a linguistic outset. Quoting Edwards (2012), one of the fathers of DP, it is described as a

systematic, empirical, and principled way of examining psychological concepts, for instance, emotion. Accordingly, the DP analyst investigates how
psychological concepts are construed in practice, and the functions of such
concepts are described as linked to their purpose in interaction. In short,
the nexus of social practices in which language is used demonstrates to the
DP analyst how psychological concepts manifest themselves (Tileagǎ and
Stokoe 2016). Classic DP studies draw on discourse-analytical terms, such
as "interpretative repertoires," and CA vocabulary, such as "membership
categorization" [the latter term derived from the lectures of Harvey Sacks
(1972, 1992)], whereas contemporary studies tend to place themselves
much more explicitly in alignment with CA, underpinning a strict empirical focus and a sequential analytical tightness.

This book is centered on practices as activities performed in social
and material settings. This means that it concentrates only occasionally
on language-related practices. Therefore, DP plays a minor role in an
overall discussion of the new framework; however, it is a great inspiration and a body of knowledge without which this book could not have
existed. Demonstrably, a different conceptualization of language and of
proficiency, as discussed in Chapters 2 and 3, can provide new insights
into LCDs as social, individual, and societal phenomena. Importantly, a
person-centered praxeology offers a tool to include QOL-related aspects
of lived disorders, including aphasia and linguistic impairment.

Analytical Implications in Applied Linguistics

This author, however, has objections to three areas of traditional pragmatic analysis of LCDs. First, within multimodal studies of LCDs, the
analytical strategy of an augmented version of CA seems to rely on the
expertise of the analyst and not on that of the participant with a disorder,
unless one agrees completely with the ontology of the EMCA program,
which states that CA is data-driven and considers the analyst to be a tech-
nician. This author finds such an analytical perspective problematic and
is seeking to come up with an alternative analytical perspective that can
address the deficit. Goodwin (2003), for instance, has demonstrated that
participants with aphasia can indeed have proficiency. However, more
problematic features of interaction with individuals with aphasia have had
very little space in the popularized EMCA studies on aphasia, including
outcomes other than successful accomplishment of meaning together
with peers, for instance, non-compliance and complaints. Second, the

status of the transcript as an analytical artefact is questioned. Third, an objection to the implicitness of the analyst's perspective is made, mainly in CA studies. The analyst seems to have gained a status of omnipotence, or at least has claimed the best possible method available so far, relying only on the next-turn proof-procedure for validation of interpretations made in the analysis of the accomplishment of the participant's meaning.

As the field of linguistics continues to grow, the number of analytical units added grows as well. The materiality of embodied interaction sheds light upon the case of observational strategies and puts the epistemology of "data" under scrutiny. Human interaction is presumed to be patterned, strategic, and structured. The presuppositions of orderliness and structure have long dominated modern applied linguistics without substantial criticism. Several issues concerning the use of "data" to uncover the mechanisms of human communication need to be scrutinized.

The Analyst as Segregationist

Traditionally, the study of the mechanisms of human interaction is based on the methodology of CA. CA's cumulative purpose is to reveal a set of micro-rules that are assumed to govern (any) human interaction. A recording and a micro-transcription are used as data in the process of analysis. These contain products that the analyst has shaped and chosen: the site, participants, and perspective. The analyst follows a strategy stepwise: first, the analyst chooses a sequence; second, the analyst characterizes which actions occur in the chosen sequence; third, the analyst describes the modes of production that the language users display. These are the conventionalized forms of "linguistic materiality" that occur in the chosen sequence and must be readable in a transcript produced by the analyst in the next step of analysis. Finally, the analyst discusses how sequential organization, timing, and turn-taking contribute to establish the participants' understandings of the meaning of the interactional actions, based on the transcript and video that the researcher entirely has produced and edited. In addition, CA raises factuality using a positivist discourse. Hence, micro-rules are characterized with expressions such as "display," "data," "account," and "demonstration" to describe cooperative meaning-making and social human agency.

The status of the analyst as expert in the omni-ordered structure of human interaction is broadly accepted in modern linguistics. CA's relentless use of a positivist vocabulary has encouraged health professionals and medical researchers to engage in interaction studies in the study of LCDs. However, too strong a positivist approach may fail to grasp important features of aphasic interaction as it is considered the prime professional practice of CA analysts to uncover the mechanisms of atypical communication such as aphasia, and limit studies of aphasia as social interaction to the accomplishment of meaning. Thus, this tendency downplays a humanist stance in the study of LCDs and develops further a positivist stance. Hence, a new analytical approach is required to initiate an assessment of development tendencies.

Segregating the Epistemology of Data

In the following, the term "data" in modern applied linguistics will be described and briefly discussed. Thereafter, a discussion of the epistemology of "data" unfolds the objections. Finally, an alternative, new analytical approach will be introduced.

Data in CA mirror sense in the making. The CA analyst considers context as created in common through interaction (Pomerantz and Fehr 1997; de Kok 2008, p. 890; Fleming 1995). The conversation is considered to be under construction (Fleming 1995, p. 92). CA analysts describe, apply, and operate a local concept of context, where focus is sat upon the interaction, including turn-taking and interaction contributions. The contributions in interaction are regarded as context-constructing units in a forward-directed time perspective (Stax 2005, p. 175). Context is within the CA framework, and, thus, defined as a sequential, interactional concept (de Kok 2008; ten Have 2007; Fleming 1997, p. 196). CA analysts have been criticized for having overfocused on the structural aspects of interaction, the structures of context, rather than focusing on the actual persons taking part and the discursive framework and settings of conversations (de Kok 2008, p. 887). Previous criticism finds that the content of the conversations studied is neglected, if not completely lost, because the mechanistic interest in sequentiality and the local context concept occupy the whole of the CA analyst's attention (de Kok 2008, p. 887; Fleming 1995, 1997).

Despite its development and application over time, the usage of the term "data" is treated as unproblematic in EMCA and CA studies. The original recordings are claimed to be the data, and transcripts are merely considered to facilitate data sessions and paraphrase data in publications. Yet, the notion of data is to be considered a result of the observer's work process and nothing else. The claim of factuality is too strong within the traditions of CA.

To put it straightforwardly, the very focus in the analysis changes when applying a person-centered praxeology. It changes from the CA perspective of observing interaction and context as a scenario where conversation takes place, to a person-centered praxeology that deals with and focuses upon the persons communicating about their understandings, verbally or non-verbally. In consequence, signs can be private signs meaningful for one individual (Harris 2009a, p. 76). Therefore, integrational analysis includes individual time-scales as well as shared time-scales and, as a result, may be conducted in a forward as well a backward perspective (temporal integration, Harris 2009a, pp. 72–73). This is not an option in traditional EMCA studies, where the analysis is always directed sequentially forward. In consequence, the history of every individual is unique (Harris 1987, p. 7), and so a person-centered praxeology indeed encourages including a lay-perspective in scientific descriptions (Pablé and Hutton 2015, pp. 50–51).

According to Harris, nothing stands for anything (Harris 1996, 1998). Sense-making is not a practice which can be made factual by multiple interpretations and supportive arguments from data sessions alone. Data sessions can help draw the researcher's attention towards certain aspects of the data. In contrast, practices are coordinated performances of private contextualization that may be traceable in, for instance, documents, video data, and transcripts, or that may not be traceable at all. Therefore, it is a key theoretical point that every contribution, including publicly available displays of understanding, is personal and structured by personal and by social relevance (Harris 2012, p. 43):

> Observers can do no more than interpret, on the basis of their individual linguistic experience, what is said or written. They may entertain no doubts about the well-foundedness of their own interpretations. But that does not automatically promote what they agree upon into an independent "fact" about the language in question.

And therefore, the forensic approach, the search for accounts and "factuality" in CA, raises a methodological problem to the integrationist (Harris 2012, p. 44):

> This gap between presupposition and demonstration, the integrationist will say, is what gives rise to the problem (…).

Moreover, this applies to both the infrastructure of the conversation examined and for the extra-situational interpretations of the analyst (Taylor and Cameron 1987). All sense-making is subject to this condition. What is being analyzed is regarded as something that has derived from the actual situation in which it was produced or otherwise demonstrated and nothing else (Harris 1996, 1998, 2009a; Harris and Wolf 2008; Ruus 1995; Hermann and Gregersen 1978). This book aims to develop an analysis which is not generating knowledge about general level patterns of social practice, but rather one that can study single trajectories through situations in the contexts in which they are found, with the purpose of being able to discuss new aspects and initiatives.

The focus in the analysis is simply different, as the analyst is not an expert in the professional practice of aphasic communication but simply an expert in describing integrational proficiency in any communication. The language makers, whether they have aphasia or not, are the experts in their own mode of communicating. This stated, it may lead to the discussion of epistemological and ontological challenges in some traditional schools in the language sciences. Additionally, if fully applied and its consequences accepted, it could lead towards a sea-change in linguistics and psychology in the status of the analyst as expert.

Earlier, the integrational discussion of data missed the opportunity of accounting for a credible, productive critique (Duncker 2011; Fleming 1995, 1997). It is this author's belief that a person-centered praxeology can incorporate an EMCA-inspired analysis and a PT approach on integrational premises. For obvious reasons, the divergences must be clarified, and the goal of the analysis must be clearly stated.

HARMONIZATION OF INTEGRATIONISM, ETHNOMETHODOLOGY AND CONVERSATION ANALYSIS

Traditional Tools for Integrational Analysis: Criticism

It is problematic that, as noted throughout Chapter 4, Harris offers IL very few analytical tools, at least from his own hand. This also applies to the integrational criticism of the presuppositions of the EMCA program (Taylor and Cameron 1987; Fleming 1995, 1997). The framework of EMCA relies on Harold Garfinkel's original idea of the pre-existence of an ever-emergent, but orderly, mechanism that manages individuals' affairs with one another: a constitutive social order (Garfinkel 1967). Members' methods are examined within EMCA, and local orders and their constitutive properties are described as a central area of interest. The general idea is to uncover how members achieve mutual understanding and how they display their actions intelligibly (Garfinkel 1967; Heritage 1984; Rawls 2008). Within EMCA, shared understanding and mutual orientation towards general rules are presupposed and linked to the core concept of "order" (Rawls 2008, p. 19):

> Garfinkel argues that what makes an action recognizable to others as an action of a particular sort are constitutive aspects of the orderliness of an action – sequential and reflexive order – that constitutes the action as a recognizable action – for this group of identified actors – engaged in just this practice together.

As presented and discussed in Chapters 2 and 4, language and human activities are considered radically indeterminate in an integrational view. IL's focus on indeterminacy is opposed to the presupposed local "orders" searched for within the EMCA program (Taylor and Cameron 1987; Hutton 2017; Zhou 2014). However, EMCA analysts would argue that locally fixed meanings are the only orders that exist, and that these are necessary for us to understand, act and engage with the world. Contrastingly, this "railing," a suitable metaphor to describe how the notion of orders is perceived within IL, as a prerequisite for individuals to exist in the world is exactly what triggers the IL critique because it inhumanely reduces humans to automata. Currently, the EMCA program is heavily criticized by Hong Kong-based integrationists, precisely for the analytical framing of EMCA. For instance, EMCA is compared to "a machine model of human behavior" (Zhou 2014, p. 1) aligned with other contemporary approaches besides IL. Christopher Hutton criticizes EMCA's analytical strategies and classifies it as "evolutionary" rather than "phenomenological" (Hutton 2017, p. 96):

> Participants experience the first-order reality of the categories and the explanatory power of their reflexive accounts, what might be termed "lived essentialism," while the external observer perceives, in "disenchanted" Weberian fashion, an ultimately contentless, although ineluctable, drive for social order (Orbuch, 1997). This suggests that classical

ethnomethodology is closer to evolutionary models of behavior than its phenomenological grounding would suggest. It is grounded in the second-order achievement of social order, as opposed to survival and reproductive success.

In similar fashion, since the 1980s, integrationists have criticized EMCA excessively for its search for regularities and structures of social action rather than intersubjectivity (Taylor and Cameron 1987, p. 161). One could argue that Hutton, in the citation given above, ascribes much will to the single individual to get things done, for instance, survival and reproductive success, by discarding the social. Yet, the social is recognized by this author in a triangulation.

Notwithstanding the orthodox Harrisian tradition of heavy criticism of all other ontologies than IL ontology, this book attempts to unfold a diffractive applied integrationism, insisting that a person-centered praxeology is operational. The fact that no integrationist has yet elaborated successfully on Harris's notion of a macrosocial component of the infrastructure of communication has led to this attempt at such an elaboration by applying IL principles in a joint analytical framework. This is methodologically inspired by EMCA in the sense that, for instance, the notion of members' methods is incorporated analytically, as well as the application of other CA-inspired vocabulary. The IL concept of macrosocial was introduced as one of three factors governing communication in Chapter 2. This author considers the macrosocial in agreement with other IL concepts. Unproblematically, some social aspects of communication and the IL concepts of contextualization and co-temporality discussed in Chapter 4 are aligned with the basis of the individualist approach this author favors, in accordance with Zhou's suggestion of a more humane linguistics (2014).

As discussed in Chapter 4, there are several overlaps between the EMCA framework and IL. Importantly, orthodox integrationists consider EMCA studies to be segregational in ontology, and they are criticized for merely replacing the system of language with a search for a system of talk (Taylor and Cameron 1987; Fleming 1995, 1997). This author, however, believes that contemporary EMCA studies, notwithstanding an interest in revealing the overall organization of talk and multimodal interaction, are so fine-tuned in their ontological considerations that a new attempt at harmonization is relevant and operational. Integrationists in the 1980s and 1990s critique that, for instance, EMCA frames a presupposed system which is explored and no longer holds. A nuance is left out in this critique, since it is the traceable consequences of talk and multimodality in interaction that are investigated, not the system organizing it. Findings are drawn from these data, not from the organizational system. Because of the historical divergence between IL and EMCA, there are inert ontological divergences in the PT–IL–EMCA approach, which are attempted to be solved by the above positioning.

The IL concept of radical indeterminacy promotes the observation that radical transitions inherently occur both in linguistic form and in the perceived meaning of actions (Orman 2017). However, these are not necessarily shared in any way and may occur implicitly as well. The observation that linguistic form and meaning radically fluctuate does not facilitate the traditional way of dealing with data. For this reason, Orman criticizes empirical sociolinguistics for being positivist (for political reasons) and for buying in on orthodox linguistics' binary of linguistic determinacy versus linguistic indeterminacy (Orman 2017). Simply, Orman argues that it is contradictory in its enterprise. By introducing IL in a PT joint framework, the rules and units from EMCA are downgraded and the role of temporality upgraded. This author, therefore, argues that the PT framing of IL–EMCA may be done as a result of a fine-tuned analysis of divergences for the purpose of the development of tools for analysis.

To the integrationist, "(t)he self-awareness of lay members is of a different order to the reflexive perspective of the ethnomethodological analyst" (Hutton 2017, p. 96). This is a key analytical difference between IL and EMCA. By pointing to this, the analyst avoids discussing the premises of contextualization and co-temporality any further, since they obviously also apply to the analyst's temporal contextualizations (Duncker 2011; Harris 1998, p. 98). In sum, this author argues that the suggested person-centered praxeology relies on a rendered ontology of language and communication in alignment with IL.

Making Indeterminacy Analyzable

Like the IL view on communication as an inherent mode of emergent human activity, Schatzki's inclination towards Heidegger's and Wittgenstein's ideas allow him to describe indeterminacy in social events (Schatzki 2013). This descriptive emergence of events and actions state an analyzable research object: the traceability of the human mode of being, becoming, and transitioning from one event to another, which is in alignment with this book. In addition, it refutes Orman's argument (2017) of the impossibility of using data other than introspection and the analyst's private speculations. Furthermore, PT promotes studies in practices, as does the EMCA program. By introducing a IL–PT ontology of indeterminacy, the problem of inclination towards a theoretical basis of determinacy in orthodox linguistics, which underlies segregational approaches, is solved.

Paradigmatic Prerequisites

Paradigmatically, EMCA draws strongly on a reformulation of sociology, while IL and PT draw on a common ground of philosophy of language and communication, which do not presuppose or highlight orientation towards "orderliness" to the same extent as EMCA. These contrasting histories of the different approaches produce diverse observations. However, these may be diffracted to turn the spotlight in empirical studies and grasp correlated, emergent practices in interaction and enrich the analysis. Therefore, this book aims to "cleanse" integrationism for criticism and reduce the area of interest to a person-centered approach concerning persons, relevant understanding, and actions, to consolidate these as the point of departure for developing a dynamic analytical perspective on understanding communication. The paradigmatic differences between CA and IL are a source of conflict (Fleming 1995, 1997). However, it is not an impossible task to discuss or to sort out language philosophically and ontologically. Rather, it is a necessity.

Aligning Integrationism with Ethnomethodology

Actual person's interactions with each other anchor the making of meaning as they go about contextualizing. The display of understandings may be considered traces of ongoing explicit contextualization. We need not document all a person demonstrates but may deal with their displays in an alternative fashion when turning the spotlight away from rule-governed social interaction and towards the concept of a person communicating what s/he contextualizes as relevant. In a person-centered approach, focus is sat on an individual and what s/he does and says instead of an interpretation of what was said and done. Simply put, the interpretation part is left out and the documentarist aspect is upgraded. This author is not convinced that social interaction is as rule-governed as supposed by the EMCA program. Therefore, orientation towards orders and rules is applied with warrants in this study (Pablé and Hutton 2015, pp. 42, 71–72; Nielsen 2011). Yet, IL is aligned with EMCA despite the latter's focus on orderliness.

Gains from Ethnomethodology

The transcriptional practices of CA make it possible for the integration-ist to paraphrase, navigate, and demonstrate experiences obtained during observation, which are reflected in the author's micro-data, conver-sations, or video data, and then to apply PT in this framing. An analy-sis on the grounds of a person-centered praxeology would then supply the CA analysis with more focus on the actual persons communicating (Goodwin 2003; Raudaskoski 2013) rather than having a fixed focus on the patterns of interaction (de Kok 2008; Fleming 1995, 1997; Harris 2009a, b). Technically, this focus is brought about by analytically apply-ing the concepts of contextualization and co-temporality. Instead of exclusively applying the categories of CA in the interpretive phase of the analysis, a base of the person-centered praxeology is founded in the persons in the situation examined. Obviously, the analysis will be carried out under new (contextualized) settings different from the situation in which the recording of the interaction was made. Due to the principle of co-temporality, time has passed (Fleming 1995, 1997; Harris 1998, 2009a; Pablé and Hutton 2015). Of course, the analysts have their own time-bound understanding of their own analysis. However, it is possible to deal with this methodological aspect by explicitly stating the analyst's ambition.

Whereas CA may have a fixed focus on tracking patterns and map-ping social interactions as so much rule-governed business, this method-ology can also be an observational point pertaining to just one amongst other infinite possible instrumentational systems of observance. A per-son-centered praxeology, on the other hand, is an alternative to a strict CA approach. In addition, it may be able to uncover new aspects of com-munication by triangulation, which might bring about a participant per-spective rather than the mere social pattern recognition that characterizes CA that adheres tightly to CA policies (Pomerantz and Fehr 1997). Furthermore, it may even account for different aspects than do analysts, who have their focus fixed on the coordination of actions and on how coordination is necessary to do things together (Wilkinson 2011, 2014; Goodwin 2000, 2003, 2013).

To clarify a point, integrationists do not just rely on private feelings. IL is very useful in combination with PT and NA. Therefore, it must be explained that the focus in this version of a person-centered praxeology is compromised but also principled by IL. The main principles applied are as mentioned above and discussed in Chapter 4: the principles of "contextualization" and "co-temporality." As such, these concepts form a person-centered praxeology. The school of integrational practices, so far, has mostly been discussed and debated as a theoretical perspective (Harris 1996, 1998; Harris and Wolf 2008; Fleming 1995; Pablé and Hutton 2015; Love 2004, 2017).

To align a person-centered praxeology with the principles of contextualization and co-temporality, the researcher already sees himself or herself as part of what is being analyzed, since introspection is part of the pragmatic approach of this perspective. It is also here that CA and integrationists part from one another. CA has a strict empirical focus whereas an integrational practice focuses, explicitly and implicitly, on the persons communicating. The transcript is thus but a token in the integrational analysis, where the wholeness of the analytical process, the original situation with the persons in it, the researcher's contextualization of his data, etc. form the actual analytical material (Duncker 2005, 2011; Nielsen 2011, 2015). The logistics of understanding are, therefore, at the center of IL analysis. To embrace the logistics of understanding and understanding as an integrational concept, a model of understanding must undergo a forensic analysis to be discussed with peers.

A Practice-Inspired Model of the Logistics of Understanding

Duncker (2005) draws the outline for an integrational practice model of communication by drawing a silhouette of the infrastructure of a communication situation and the persons communicating in it (see Fig. 5.1). The model contains multiparty communication with the illustration of a possible sequence of initiative: A, and a following response: B and C, delivered in consequence of A, and D, not directed towards A, yet situated within this sociomaterial setting.

The model demonstrates the intention of the initiator and represents the interlocutor's following possible actions and responses. All participants, intentions, responses, interpretations, and coordination are being governed by the principles of Harris's three factors: B—biomechanical; M—macrosocial; and Ct—circumstantial (Duncker 2005, pp. 141–142; Harris 1998, p. 25). Referring to these factors, Duncker points to the

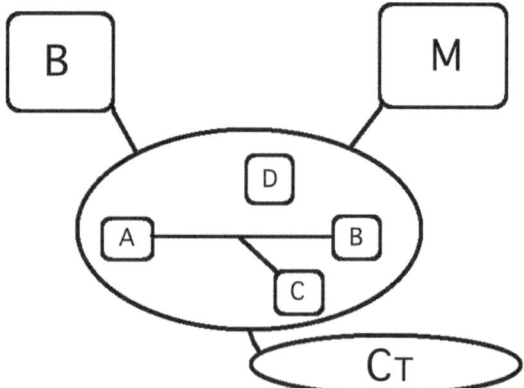

Fig. 5.1 This author's simplified version of Duncker's model

potential of dismissing traditional models of communication and adapting the integrational model with which she enhances the influence of new observations and new observational points for the analyst. Concepts such as misunderstandings will, Duncker argues, be considered normal and may even contribute to the development of a new approach to investigate the dynamics of communicational processes with an integrational model of communication (Duncker 2005, p. 143).

The person-centered praxeology which this book supports does not draw only on the directly observable; therefore, it cannot be categorized strictly as an empirical approach to human interaction, as is the CA approach to human interaction. The CA analyst uncovers the various strategies applied by the participants communicatively. It is, however, presupposed that participants do display understandings (Sacks et al. 1974, p. 729). Also, it is presupposed that participants in the next turn display their understandings of their own previous turn or of other participants' turns displayed in previous turns. As noted by Garfinkel, the focus is on what the participants in situations deem necessary to "reveal," though they might be thinking of many other things about what is going on, but if they do not make a point about them to the other party, then it is a case of "letting it pass" (Garfinkel 1967, p. 3). This forward-directed interpretive method is supposed to account for understandings and to supply the "proof" for the analyst's interpretation of the participants' understandings in talk-in-action (Sacks et al. 1974, p. 729). This argument is supported by Fleming, who emphasizes that Sacks and his fellow analysts themselves originally stated that the organization of turn-taking is their case and not "the particular outcome in particular settings" (Sacks cited by Fleming 1997, p. 199). In a person-centered praxeology, on this ground, attention is drawn to the integrational perception of the logistics of communicational situations, as demonstrated in the integrational model of communication by Duncker (2005).

The mechanisms of conversations that CA seeks to uncover and map systematically (Sacks et al. 1974) are only used as navigational tools by the person-centered praxeology. Displayed meaning-making is thus demonstrated partially and accounted for analytically using CA strategies. The participants' integrational proficiencies are in focus and these are not measured by their productiveness in the interaction or dialogue per se. Moreover, their proficiency is revealed by their attempts to and ability to integrate themselves, and only partially by coordinating in the situation with interlocutors and the material setting. As noted by Fleming (1997, p. 203), this does not align sequentiality with co-temporality, since co-temporality also embraces simultaneity. We are not governed by the clockwise sequentiality of CA in real life; we are language makers and we make up language as we go. Fleming (1997) and Duncker (2004) agree that an integrational rhetoric would account for a "radical contextualization" (Fleming 1997, p. 205), meaning that an analysis of human acts attends to particular situations and is distributed over time. In short, the rigidness of CA's sequential organization of the analysis rooted in the next turn proof procedure must be abandoned to study a participant perspective founded in empirically situated discursive action (Fleming 1997, p. 207).

THE NEW PROGRAM FOR A PERSON-CENTERED PRAXEOLOGY

The general observation list below, inspired by Schegloff and Sacks' programs, is an idea catalogue that states areas for the advancement of a person-centered praxeology. It proposes situations in which contributions can be made to advance the establishment of and increase in closer observations of situational interactions in future studies:

1. observations of speakers/observation of agency;
2. actions as single or simultaneous occurrences;
3. observation of action transition from one situation to another;
4. topic trajectories from one situation to another;
5. material trajectories from one situation to another;
6. intra-situational order: continuous/discontinuous local event;

7. extra-situational event order: initiation/continuer of previous event;
8. action constructional units employed;
9. situational constructional units employed;
10. repair: errors/violations of the employment of semiotic resources.

Overall, these are to be considered:

- Areas for observing what happens
- Traceability tools
- Trans-situational tools
- After/retro-contextualization tools
- Anti-criticism of EMCA
- A prioritizing of PT
- A new assessment standard of social interaction with LCDs.

A unique focus on troubles is foregrounded in this book's investigation and data analysis. Typical interactional sources of trouble in rehabilitation and intervention practices include compliance and non-compliance, emotions and requests unmet, cases of direct persuasion, and, most often, complaints. Traditionally, complaints and the above cases have been studied within CA in sequential analyses (Drew 1998; Heinemann and Traverso 2009; Heinemann 2009; Jefferson 1988). These demonstrate fine-tuned analyses of participant orientation towards one another. However, in an integrational perspective, categories are too solid to capture the contextual nuances of a more person-centered approach. The attempt is thus to consolidate a person-centered approach through an elaboration of traditional methods in a practice frame.

REFERENCES

Barad, K. (2007). *Meeting the universe halfway: Quantum physics and the entanglement of matter and meaning.* Durham, NC: Duke University Press.

Conrad, C. (2011). Forståelseshandlingen: En empirisk afprøvet teori om narrativ forståelse som situeret betydning i dannelse. PhD dissertation, Københavns Universitet, København.

de Kok, C. (2008). The role of context in conversation analysis: Reviving an interest in ethno-methods. *Journal of Pragmatics, 40*(5), 886–903.

Drew, P. (1998). Complaints about transgression and misconduct. *Research on Language and Social Interaction, 31,* 295–325.

Duncker, D. (2004). Som at gå i Jesus' fodspor. In M. Rathje & L. Svenstrup (Eds.), *Sprogpsykologi - udvalgte kerneemner* (pp. 201–220). København: Museum Tusculanum.

Duncker, D. (2005). Den integrerende kommunikationsmodel. In P. Widell & M. Kunøe (Eds.), *10. møde om udforskningen af dansk sprog* (pp. 137–146). Aarhus: Fællestrykkeriet for Sundhedsvidenskab og Humaniora Aarhus Universitet.

Duncker, D. (2011). On the empirical challenge to integrational studies in language. *Language Sciences, 33*(4), 533–543.

Edwards, D. (2012). Discursive and scientific psychology. *British Journal of Social Psychology, 51*(3), 425–435.

Fleming, D. (1995). The search for an integrational account of language: Roy Harris and conversation analysis. *Language Sciences, 17*(1), 73–98.

Fleming, D. (1997). Is ethnomethodological conversation analysis an "integrational" account of language? In G. Wolf & N. Love (Eds.), *Linguistics inside out* (pp. 182–207). Amsterdam: John Benjamins.

Garfinkel, H. (1967). *Studies in ethnomethodology.* Englewood Cliffs, NJ: Prentice Hall.

Glintborg, C. (2015). Disabled and not normal. *Narrative Inquiry, 25*(1), 1–22.

Glintborg, C. (Ed.). (2018). *Rehabiliteringspsykologi: En introduktion i teori og praksis.* Aarhus: Aarhus Universitetsforlag.

Goodwin, C. (2000). Action and embodiment within human interaction. *Journal of Pragmatics, 32,* 1489–1522.

Goodwin, C. (2003). Conversational frameworks for the accomplishment of meaning in aphasia. In C. Goodwin (Ed.), *Conversation and brain damage* (pp. 90–116). Oxford: Oxford University Press.

Goodwin, C. (2013). The co-operative, transformative organization of human action and knowledge. *Journal of Pragmatics, 46*(1), 8–23.

Harris, R. (1981). *The language myth.* London: Duckworth.

Harris, R. (1987). *The language machine.* Ithaca, NY: Cornell University Press.

Harris, R. (1996). *Signs, language and communication.* London: Routledge.

Harris, R. (1998). *Introduction to integrational linguistics.* Oxford: Pergamon.

Harris, R. (2009a). *Integrationist notes and papers 2006–2008.* Gamlingay: A Bright Pen.

Harris, R. (2009b). *After epistemology.* Gamlingay: A Bright Pen.

Harris, R. (2012). *Integrationist notes and papers 2012.* Gamlingay: A Bright Pen.

Harris, R., & Wolf, G. (Eds.). (2008). *Integrational linguistics: A first reader.* Oxford: Pergamon.

Heinemann, T. (2009). Participation and exclusion in third party complaints. *Journal of Pragmatics, 41*(12), 2435–2451.

Heinemann, T., & Traverso, V. (2009). Complaining in interaction. *Journal of Pragmatics, 41*(12), 2381–2384.

Heritage, J. (1984). *Garfinkel and ethnomethodology.* Oxford: Basil Blackwell.

Hermann, J., & Gregersen, F. (1978). *Gennem sproget; om undersøgelse af sprogbrug i samfundet.* København: Gyldendal.

Hutton, C. (2017). The self and the "monkey selfie": Law, integrationism and the nature of the first order/second order distinction. *Language Sciences, 61,* 93–103.

Jefferson, G. (1988). On the sequential organization of troubles-talk in ordinary conversation. *Social Problems, 35*(4), 418–441.

Larsen, M., & Raudaskoski, P. (2016). Medieret diskursanalyse og neksusanalyse. In A. Horsbøl & P. Raudaskoski (Eds.), *Diskurs og praksis: Teori, metode og analyse* (pp. 89–109). København: Samfundslitteratur.

Legg, C., & Penn, P. (2013). Uncertainty, vulnerability, and isolation: Factors framing quality of life with aphasia in a South African township. In N. Warren & L. Manderson (Eds.), *Reframing disability and quality of life: A global perspective* (pp. 17–37). Dordrecht: Springer.

Love, N. (2004). Cognition and the language myth. Distributed cognition and integrational linguistics. *Language Sciences, 26*(6), 525–544.

Love, N. (2017). On languaging and languages. *Language Sciences, 61,* 1–35.

Nicolini, D. (2012). *Practice theory, work, and organization: An introduction.* Oxford: Oxford University Press.

Nielsen, C. (2011). Towards applied integrationism: Integrating autism in teaching and coaching sessions. *Language Sciences, 33*(4), 593–602.

Nielsen, C. (2015). Senhjerneskade i et forståelsesperspektiv. In S. Frimann, M. Sørensen, & H. Wentzer (Eds.), *Sammenhænge i sundhedskommunikation* (pp. 247–281). Aalborg: Aalborg Universitetsforlag.

Orman, J. (2017). Indeterminacy in sociolinguistics and integrationist theory. In A. Pablé (Ed.), *Critical humanist perspectives: The integrational turn in philosophy of language and communication* (pp. 96–113). London: Routledge.

Pablé, A., & Hutton, C. (2015). *Signs, meaning and experience.* Berlin: De Gruyter Mouton.

Pomerantz, A., & Fehr, J. B. (1997). Conversation analysis: An approach to the study of social action as sense-making practices. In T. van Dijk (Ed.), *Discourse as social interaction* (pp. 64–91). Thousand Oaks, CA: Sage.

Raudaskoski, P. (2013). From understanding to participation: A relational approach to embodied practices. In T. Keisanen, E. Kärkkäinen, M. Rauniomaa, P. Siitonen, & M. Siromaa (Eds.), *Multimodal discourses of participation, AFinLA yearbook* (Vol. 71, pp. 103–121). Jyväskylä: Suomen Soveltavan Kielitieteen Yhdistyks (AFinLA).

Rawls, A. (2008). Quoted in editor's introduction. In H. Garfinkel (Ed.), *Toward a sociological theory of information* (pp. 1–100). Boulder, CO: Paradigm Publishers.

Reckwitz, A. (2002). Towards a theory of social practices: A development in culturalist theorizing. *European Journal of Social Theory, 5*(2), 243–263.

Ruus, H. (1995). *Danske kerneord* (Vol. 1, pp. 3–18). København: Museum Tusculanum.

Sacks, H. (1972). An initial investigation of the usability of conversational data for doing sociology. In D. Sudnow (Ed.), *Studies in social interaction* (pp. 31–74). New York: Free Press.

Sacks, H. (1992). *Lectures on conversation* (Vols. 1–2). Oxford: Basil Blackwell.

Sacks, H., Schegloff, E., & Jefferson, G. (1974). A simplest systematics for the organization of turn-taking for conversation. *Language, 50*(4), 696–735.

Schatzki, T. (2013). Activity as an indeterminate social event. In S. Reynolds, D. Egan, & A. Weneland (Eds.), *Wittgenstein and Heidegger: Pathways and provocations* (pp. 179–194). London: Routledge.

Scollon, R. (2001). *Mediated discourse: The nexus of practice* (pp. 1–18). New York: Routledge.

Scollon, R., & Scollon, S. W. (2004). *Discourse and the emerging internet.* London: Routledge.

Scollon, R., & Scollon, S. W. (2007). Nexus analysis: Refocusing ethnography on action. *Journal of Sociolinguistics, 11*(5), 608–625.

Stax, T. (2005). Samtaler i detaljer, detaljer i samtalen. In M. Jarvinen & N. Mik-Meyer (Eds.), *Kvalitative metoder i et interaktionistisk perspektiv* (pp. 169–190). København: Hans Reitzels Forlag.

Taylor, T., & Cameron, D. (1987). *Analysing conversation: Rules and units in the structure of talk.* Oxford: Pergamon Press.

ten Have, P. (2007). *Doing conversation analysis.* Thousand Oaks, CA: Sage Publications.

Tileagă, C., & Stokoe, E. (2016). *Discursive psychology: Classic and contemporary issues.* London: Routledge.

Toolan, M. (1996). *Total speech: An integrational linguistic approach to language.* Durham, NC: Duke University Press.

Wallace, S., Worrall, L., Rose, T., Dorze, G., Isaksen, J., Pak, A., et al. (2016). Which outcomes are most important to people with aphasia and their families? An international nominal group technique study framed within the ICF. *Disability and Rehabilitation, 39*(14), 1–16.

Warren, N., & Manderson, L. (2013). Reframing disability and quality of life: Contextual nuances. In N. Warren & L. Manderson (Eds.), *Reframing disability and quality of life: A global perspective* (pp. 1–16). Dordrecht: Springer.

Wiggins, S., & Potter, J. (2007). Discursive psychology. In C. Willig & W. Stainton-Rogers (Eds.), *The Sage handbook of qualitative research in psychology* (pp. 73–90). Thousand Oaks, CA: Sage.

Wilkinson, R. (2011). Changing interactional behavior: Using conversation analysis in intervention programmes for aphasic conversation. In C. Antaki (Ed.), *Applied conversation analysis: Intervention and change in institutional talk* (pp. 32–53). Basingstoke: Palgrave Macmillan.

Wilkinson, R. (2014). Research on language and social interaction intervening with conversation analysis in speech and language therapy: Improving aphasic conversation intervening with conversation analysis in speech and language therapy. *Research on Language and Social Interaction, 47*(3), 219–238.

World Health Organization. (1995). *WHOQOL–100.* Division of Mental Health. Geneva: World Health Organization.

Zhou, F. (2014). *System, order, creativity: Models of the human in the twentieth-century linguistic theories.* PhD dissertation, University of Hong Kong, Hong Kong.

CHAPTER 6

Probing the New Analytical Perspective

Abstract The outline for a person-centered praxeology takes its point of departure in the methodological framing of zooming in and zooming out (Nicolini in Organ Stud 30:1391–1418, 2009), as discussed in Chapter 5. The zooming-in part combines the approaches of integrational linguistics and ethnomethodology and conversation analysis methodologically. Zooming in traces significant trajectories across excerpts, whereas zooming out describes larger frames of practices. Building upon the discussion from previous chapters, the pros and cons of combining analytical concepts are discussed. The analytical framework in this chapter is presented along with video data. Frames of practices are unfolded in order to establish a base on which to inform professional practice about their social consequences. An abductive element of the analytical strategy is given attention and scrutinized.

Keywords Person-centeredness · Processuality
Participant perspective · Traceability · Scrutiny

INCLUSION AND EXCLUSION AS DISCURSIVE PRACTICES

This chapter combines integrational linguistics (IL) and ethnomethodology and conversation analysis program (EMCA) in a joint practice theory (PT) framework. The overall aim is to add an IL ontological

© The Author(s) 2018   95
C. M. B. Klemmensen, *Integrating the Participants' Perspective
in the Study of Language and Communication Disorders*,
https://doi.org/10.1007/978-3-319-78634-6_6

twist to existing EMCA–PT methodologies of processual meaning-making. As discussed throughout this book, IL has little presence as an applied science; therefore, this text is a first step towards an IL-inspired analysis of language and communication disorder (LCDs). Analytically, the attempt is to investigate practices of inclusion and exclusion while probing the IL person-centered concept of contextualization in an inter-action analysis. Since very little applied IL tradition exists in language disorders (Nielsen 2011, 2015), this analysis is inspired by analytical tra-ditions in bordering fields. Two currents serve as the main inspirations to investigate situated inclusion and exclusion: interaction studies in aphasia and, more generally, studies of social activity and multimodality. Here, the traditions of the inspirational sources are unfolded further.

First, this analysis is inspired by interaction studies. Specifically, data-driven approaches to individuals with aphasia's participatory opportuni-ties in interaction are an inspiration. As discussed in Chapters 3 and 5, within that field, studies have focused on the co-construction of turns, on accomplishing meaning together, and on gesturing as *semiotic resource* (Goodwin 2000, 2013). Analysts of aphasic discourse in interaction have developed a threefold understanding of this type of communication (Goodwin 2003; Perkins 2003; Wilkinson 2011; Legg and Penn 2013; Wallace et al. 2016):

1. Characterize aphasia as an atypical form of interaction (e.g., Antaki and Wilkinson 2013);
2. Focus on the organization of repair in interaction (e.g., Perkins 2003); and
3. Develop supportive communicative strategies for peers in interac-tion (e.g., Wilkinson 2011).

Second, this analysis is inspired by general studies in social activity. In recent years, this course of study has evolved. Namely, the visual turn in multimodality has moved interaction studies away from logocen-trism (McIlvenny 1995; Mondada 2016, p. 336) and towards action. In sum, a shift of priority from talk in traditional EMCA to embodiment (Nevile 2015) and materiality (Raudaskoski 1999) marks multimodality. Cumulative CA notions on embodiment and materiality have enhanced the emphasis on the role of materiality in interaction,[1] which has embed-ded this tradition with a range of new areas to study, including:

- The use of objects in social activity (Raudaskoski 1999; Mondada 2014);
- The spatiality of social activity (Goodwin 2000; Mondada 2014; Scollon and Scollon 2004);
- The temporality of social activity (Mondada 2014; Middleton and Brown 2005); and
- The haptic organization of social activity (Goodwin 2017; Cekaite 2016).

These are noteworthy inspirations for this investigation. Yet, EMCA and multimodality share similar features: The analysis is sequentially organized, and the next-turn proof-procedure analytically accounts for the intersubjective reception of action (Mondada 2016, p. 360).

Resemiotization

The notion of *resemiotization*, coined by Rick Iedema (2003), is a third analytical inspiration. It serves the investigative purpose of tracing activities and their consequences across iterative frames of social activities. Basically, Iedema's resemiotization is about *historizing meaning* (Iedema 2003, p. 40). This affords a more fine-tuned analysis of larger frames of processuality (i.e., socio-material meaning-making over time and across situations). Furthermore, it aids in tracing two layers of progress and the transformation of meaning. First, it traces the course of social action found in local talk. Second, this conceptual idea tracks how such courses transform from local talks into documents following institutional and cultural habits, which generate categorical consequences. For instance, it shows that Hugh Mehan's work (1993) demonstrates how a teacher's perception of a child's behavior transforms into a clinical diagnosis through a process of exosomatic translations. In sum, Iedema investigates local interactions and shows how they may transform into ritualized ways of thinking and acting over time (Iedema 2003, p. 42).

However, resemiotization is based on the common linguistic idea of decoding, encoding, and recoding signs, which account for the transformation of meaning. Meaning, as an IL concept, is strictly experiential and grounded in individual contextualization (Harris 2009a, p. 71). Yet, this author finds resemiotization promising as a way to analytically trace the development of action. In this analysis, resemiotization is applied within an IL-inspired analytical approach.[2]

A Broader Understanding of Practices with Language Disorders

More generally, the aim of this book's analytical approach is to contribute to a broader understanding of lived language disorders, such as aphasia, building upon the above inspirations. However, while EMCA, multimodality, and Iedema's resemiotization focus on the scenario of social activity, this book draws on the IL approach to meaning. In this approach, meaning is conceptualized as radically indeterminate as it is centered in a person's historical body and what s/he experiences in interaction, explicitly or implicitly, and, in many ways, is aligned with PT[3] (Orman 2017; Schatzki 2013; Scollon and Scollon 2004, 2007).

ANALYTICAL POSITIONING

This author affiliates with what is conceptualized as a Danish version of IL (Duncker 2005, 2011; Nielsen 2011, 2015; Conrad 2011; Worsøe 2014; Damm 2016). Prevalently, Danish IL studies compromise IL orthodoxy and favor probing applied aspects of IL—an approach gaining ground in Europe and gaining appreciation outside of it (Pablé and Hutton 2015). Shifting to an IL-inspired ontology in the study of social activity provides an invitation to foreground agency within praxeology by introducing a person-centered perspective. This author's positioning is entangled with her research motivation, specifically:

- to pay more attention to interactional consequences with aphasia in rehabilitation;
- to inform clinical practice and policy-makers by giving a voice to the voiceless; and
- to reduce emotional distress with LCDs and acquired brain injury (ABI).

The aim of this study is to contribute to support a reduction of emotional distress in interaction for individuals with aphasia and ABI. Convincingly, these points translate into the three steps of Ron Scollon and Suzie Scollon's (2004) suggestion for Nexus analysis (NA), discussed in Chapters 2 and 5. Their *Fieldguide* (Scollon and Scollon 2004, pp. 152–178) includes: Navigating, engaging, and possibly changing practices. These guidelines fit this author's consideration that aphasia and ABI are under-studied as social issues (Scollon and Scollon 2004, p. 153; Parr 2008).

Crucially, Hester Parr (2008, p. 20) discusses the taboo in Western societies that is social marginalization. Investigating the social exclusion of individuals with chronic illness and disability, Parr points to Pamela Moss and Isabel Dyck's (2003) argument that chronic illness and disability are unappreciated by "not only social theorists, but by the state, family, colleagues, insurers […]" (Parr 2008, p. 21) for their indefiniteness and flux qualities. In other words, language deficiency and brain injury are difficult social themes and not necessarily prestigious research. The desired outcome from this study is to emphasize these themes by engaging in relevant discussions on the topic of social marginalization. In sum, this book, together with a line of other researchers, aims at informing quality of life (QOL) practices (Wallace et al. 2016; Saldert et al. 2015).

Theorizing Practices Practiced: Human Action

The exploration of practices at different levels is characterized by *shifting theoretical lenses* (Nicolini 2009, p. 1391). Basically, this maneuver of changing the analytical perspective with the acts of zooming in and out allows the analyst to consider complementary sides of phenomena. As recounted in Chapters 2, 3, and 4, IL perspective addresses the three integrational factors that govern all communication (Harris 1998, p. 29): the biomechanical, the macrosocial, and the circumstantial factors, are considered entangled. This entanglement perspective invites the opportunity to explore analysis at different levels.

In this view, a person-centered perspective is conceptualized as the entanglement of individual, social, and situational configurations: Physiology, materiality, psychology, human action, linguistic actions, extra-linguistic actions, and multimodality combined frame this interaction analysis. Relevant local displays or ecological details may be foregrounded, or they may be considered part of a wider circumference linked to the broader meaning of an action (Scollon and Scollon 2004, p. 171), depending on what is being done and oriented to circumstantially.

In similar fashion, Charles Goodwin (2018) conceptualizes a broad concept of human action as constituted by the ability to work *co-operatively* (Goodwin 2018, p. 3). Human action is considered a product of cultural practice. Significantly, humans act together by interacting, literally building on one another's actions. This co-working-in-action functions by the decomposition and reuse of materials, whether semiotic or physical materials, which accumulate and constitute the exchange of knowledge that is produced when humans act together. Goodwin applies the notion of *lamination* to grasp "the different kinds of structure that participants draw upon to build action in concert with each other" (2013, p. 12).[4] In short, practices are regarded co-constituted through the process of social activity, where we constantly "inhabit each other's actions" (Goodwin 2013, p. 8; 2018, p. 11). In this view, moral and social responsibility are topicalized in human cooperative action.

The Organization of Analyzing Practices and Their Consequences

The visibility of the complexity of practice is investigated through video analysis (Jordan and Henderson 1995, p. 79). The iterative stream of actions being co-elaborated demonstrate a therapeutic idea of the properties of human social proficiency. This analysis contributes to the understanding of the social consequences of aphasia and ABI, with a significant account for an individual's integrational proficiency. First, the video ethnographic study is introduced. Then, a macrosocial discourse analysis zooms out (Nicolini 2009) integrating discourse orders and organizational discursivity before the situated analysis. Next, situated actions in local interaction are investigated by zooming in (Nicolini 2009) to capture phenomena emerging from the flow of situated indeterminacy contrasted with the social accomplishment of determinacy. In this analytical probing, this processuality is investigated as entangled rather than as counter positions.

Towards a Person-Centered Praxeology

An Idiographic Single Case Study

This section introduces the study's empirical data. The study was conducted using video ethnography, and recordings were made with individuals with aphasia and severe ABI. In the fall of 2012, Professor Pirkko Raudaskoski, Assistant Professor Antonia Krummheuer, and this author began a series of ethnographic video visits to a residential care facility primarily for phase 4 individuals.[5] *Phase 4* means that the person no longer qualifies for treatment at the hospital and is categorized as being at the end of treatment. This idiographic analysis centers on the social conditions of a phase 4 individual.

The data excerpts are of a male individual at this permanent care facility. He is in his forties with ABI after trauma twenty years earlier. Clinically, he has aphasia, sensory disturbances in one side of the body, is partially paralyzed, and experiences spasticity. In consequence, he uses a wheelchair to move around. Cognitively, he has memory deficiency and is considered cognitively challenged. Apart from these clinical details, his identity and the place he lives are protected and anonymized. Hereafter, he is referred to as *Søren* for acquaintance purposes. Informed consent was given and restated for this study, including consent from legal guardians. No restrictions were placed on the participation in this study. In this analysis, a collection of our case participant's contributions and his responses in social settings are traced in video recordings forming a trajectory of incidents. Two examples serve as the core data (ten Have 2004, pp. 126–132).

Trajectories of Inclusion and Exclusion

This study maps trajectories of inclusion and exclusion in specific participatory practices involving our case participant. Participatory practices were observed, analyzed, and assessed as an embedded matter of social interaction. Practices were conceptualized in a participant perspective (Nielsen 2015, p. 261). The analysis follows specific circumstantial traits and patterns in order to account for and discuss their consequences.

The aim of this study is to demonstrate traceable communicative routines. The excerpts have common themes in infrastructure, either verbally or communicatively. To construct situational frames, vocabulary from praxeological studies, as well as integrational terms, are applied to demonstrate how our case participant is constructed and deconstructed as abled versus disabled. This is done to describe local practices of inclusion versus exclusion and cultural discrepancies.

This author sought to approach and grasp the relational connections between this individual and others in specific settings and to analyze these entanglements. The project focused on the communicative patterns of inclusion and exclusion, especially on how the expected and actual troubles are oriented to and were attempted to be solved. The traceability of such complex trajectories recurring in and across situations was a focus in this investigation (Nicolini 2012; Scollon and Scollon 2004).

- What kind of answers may be sought in the complex configuration of trajectories?
- How is it possible to account for such complexity and for the consequences of entangled complexity?

To answer these questions, traceability has been foregrounded in the organization of the data set. The practice framing of the analysis leads towards the idea of situational analysis (Clarke 2005), which takes its point of departure in complexity and various entanglements of practices practiced in a specific setting with specified participants. Situational analysis is not applied explicitly in this account but serves as an associated founding idea.

This study refocuses on the psychosocial consequences in interaction for the individual. The participant's impairments were not the theoretical point of departure but a social consequence found in interaction. This small change of focus aligns the analysis with the international classification of functioning, disability and health (ICF) model's QOL conceptualization of inclusion practices as it focuses on the individual's experience with language disorders. The local ecology of the situation entails the circumstantial factors in configuration with biomechanical and macrosocial factors governing the way in which the communication unfolds when using a person-centered approach to the data. Starting from a person-centered praxeology, a phenomenological stance is taken. Contrastingly, studies in atypical interaction describe and analyze language disorders and disability, starting from the social constitution of the impairment rather than the individual experience of it. Possibly, findings derived with other abled-focused perspectives result in divergent conclusions. However, this person-centered approach singles out the contextualized praxeological configuration of one person.

Video Recording and Technology for Qualitative Analysis

Over thirty hours of video recordings were made at approximately two-weekly intervals over three months, and followed up by several visits where the site and its participants were investigated further. The recordings were configurations from several cameras (i.e., still, wearable, GoPro, and steady cameras), which produced multiangle recordings. GoPro cameras were attached to the researchers' chests or heads, and the still cameras, steady-cams, and GoPro cameras were distributed in the room to access a variety of views. GoPro cameras form the transcripts presented as data references in this analysis.

Initial Data Elaboration

This analysis draws on the author's archive of clip collections accumulated in the video ethnographic program Transana™. This software serves to manage data and for initiating video analysis. Transana™ is embedded with tools for organizing recordings in libraries. Clip tools are used for coding the material. Quick Clips and Standard Clips are the basic analytical units which are applied to organize collections. The structure of collections serves as a qualitative methodology in the sense that keywords, snapshots, and clips can be organized in certain ways that help form a theoretical understanding of the data. The further technicalities will not be discussed in this book. Importantly, the software helps the analyst transform raw video data into theory. This author has been engaged with the videos since 2012. The recordings have been elaborated by selection and coding, mainly using the tool clip collections. Several video clips were stored in an archive with thematic headlines, which organized the data and formed an analytical basis. This adds to the development of analysis as it invites the analyst to continue thematic noticing (Laurier 2014a). The compilation of clips from the main video source give an overview of relevant themes. These are elaborated by adding notes and transcripts, which generate comparative noticing. The clips are organized under themes and by keywords and are embedded with the analyst's notes on conflicts, expression of emotion, memory, etc. As a video analytical tool, Transana™ enables handling large amounts of data, quick navigation, and gives an extensive overview of the trajectories of content that is made available by the coding tools.

Selection of Excerpts for Analysis

Importantly, as noted by Charles Antaki et al. (2003), despite ongoing discussion within the field, discourse analysts rarely distinguish where theory starts and when method ends. This author will, however, attempt to track the process from the selection of excerpts to the final production of excerpts presented in the analysis. Two examples are drawn from this author's data archive. The interactional consequences and the processuality of the social activities are traced in the videos and followed in new participant recordings.

Video Analyst's Paradox

Video analysis is a professional practice, like other interpretive practices, which has its own logics-in-use (Sarangi 2007, p. 569). These excerpts, thus, represent a research process. The excerpts have been processed through the course of numerous phases. Together, the activities of detailed inspections of the material, participation in data sessions, presentations in research communities, and discussions with researchers have generated this author's perception of the material (Laurier 2014a). The excerpts are, thus, beyond the process of transcription, embedded with expert's knowledge. Furthermore, this author's understanding is afforded by this process, which has drawn her attention to noticing distinct aspects of the working environment of the data. These are now foregrounded, whereas others are given less attention, in accordance with her research motivation and ambition.

An eclectic strategy for accomplishing coherency is necessary to account for and communicate the practices at work (Nicolini 2012, p. 213). Points both relevant and irrelevant to this final analysis have been noted during the recording and later during research activity. Notes relevant to localizing the nexus of practice have been selected, elaborated, and used for gathering further knowledge on the investigation of the practices at work in the excerpts. Notes were taken during and after the recording episodes, added during the review of the recorded material in Transana™ when clips were selected and added in collections, and added during new selection phases in data sessions and after conference presentations. In format, the excerpts themselves represent a process of resemiotization (Iedema 2003; Laurier 2014a), since the excerpt formatting combines the recordings and the accumulated notes, transcripts, discussions, and their reformatting, to make up the present data. The excerpts are, thus, embedded within a resemiotization process. Furthermore, the cycles of discourses circulating the data have been researched both during and after the initial selection of the excerpts.

The transcription of the excerpts was done by this author and assessed by peer researchers. The technique for peer assessment was showing anonymized video excerpts and presenting transcribed sequences of the videos using simple Jeffersonian transcription conventions (Sacks et al. 1974, pp. 731–733). These were later supplemented with multimodal annotations authored by Charles Goodwin (2018, pp. 19–20; Goodwin et al. 2012), and Lorenza Mondada (2014, 2016). Orthographic supplements have been added to communicate the multimodal details in a more fine-tuned way, which came to this author's attention as a result of the process of noticing with video analysis (Laurier 2014a; Jordan and Henderson 1995).

Pictorial Data Representation

In this analysis, the video excerpts were presented by multimodal micro-transcription and by images of interactants. Visualizations were based on screenshots which had been anonymized by this author. Finally, screenshots of the material setting were presented. Pictorial material was included to scaffold the step-by-step, visually inspired analysis (Laurier 2014b; Mondada 2016), and to give the reader a sense of time and space frames. This also allowed for an analysis conducted sideways, instead of from above, and to follow the trajectories of practices.

ZOOMING OUT

Becoming a Patient with Aphasia and ABI

In order to consider the importance of social consequences of aphasia and ABI, social framing tools from NA were introduced. A fine-tuned analysis of the local constructions of aphasia and ABI recurring in the data involves the inclusion of wider circumferences of action, timescales, and cycles of discourse in order to locate the nexus of practice (Scollon and Scollon 2004, pp. 148–154; 2007, p. 615). Therefore, this idiographic analysis used large-scale zooming out. Zooming out means "trailing practices and their connections" (Nicolini 2012, p. 228). In this study, zooming out was applied in three movements conceptualizing:

1. the typical process of becoming a resident in a permanent care home;
2. the study site and significant aspects of its ecology; and
3. the inclusion policies of this place.

To follow connections, the zooming out starts at the point of acquiring a stroke or a trauma. Then, the process towards becoming a phase 4 resident at a residential care facility is described. *Circumferencing*(Scollon and Scollon 2004, p. 171) medical history and discourses at the site of engagement gives meaning to the investigation of particular actions. Furthermore, significant circumferences serve as analytical resources to assess a case participant's integrational proficiency. Therefore, several theoretical lenses were applied in this analysis.

First Circumference: Becoming a Resident at a Permanent Care Center

This journey starts with fast pace, and it ends with a sense of timelessness (Nielsen 2015, p. 247). Indeed, the transitions are a journey from being hospitalized after trauma or stroke to receiving a diagnosis of ABI. This was true for our case participant in the care facility.

At the point of hospitalization, the clinical damage is assessed and evaluated. Hereafter, immediate lifesaving treatment is initiated. In the beginning, the patient is continuously assessed by health professionals at the hospital. During the process of treatment, the patient transitions from needing immediate attention to being able to manage basic tasks. Typically, the patient is transferred to a specialized rehabilitation center a few weeks after trauma. Still, the patient is under constant observation and treatment plans are created and updated continuously. Once the patient is stabilized, rehabilitation comes into focus as the main activity. As the patient moves from one phase to the next, progress is registered. New initiatives are discussed with the patient and their care team along recovery. Once the patient can manage everyday tasks, s/he is ready to return to home. In the case of severe impairments after trauma, little or no progress emerges during the months of rehabilitation. In this case, the patient is reassessed, rated, and categorized. Treatment is ended without the patient reaching recovery. These cases are categorized as phase 4 cases when there is little or no chance for further improvement following hospitalization, medical treatment, and rehabilitation. Persons who are categorized as phase 4 are considered stable but not cured. In addition, these individuals require lifelong care and attention at different levels. Accordingly, the local law regulates how society treats and engages with individuals who have impairments. Since 2007, the rehabilitation of individuals with ABI in Denmark has been decentralized to local governments and municipalities, meaning that. acce to services varies from region to region. Psychologically, emotional and identity disturbances are registered after treatment, rather than rehabilitation (Glintborg 2015). There are, however, standards being developed at a political level for how inclusion should be implemented. For some individuals with acquired impairments, spending the rest of their life in a residential care facility is an inevitable option. Politically, it is suggested that individuals are socially included regardless of their physical or cognitive impairments. Unfortunately, individuals with ABI are more than likely to be excluded from societal everyday life.

Second Circumference: The Nexus of Practice

This section describes the site of the recordings. Significant details and policies of the place are taken into consideration when approaching local interactions and understanding local practices. The study site serves as a residential care facility for individuals who are diagnosed with moderate to severe brain injury. It offers residence for individuals with ABI in private rooms. Specifically, the care home has twenty-two apartments for ABI phase 4 individuals and two rehabilitation apartments. Several technological, pedagogical, and training facilities are available on site. Each individual is rated in three categories to determine whether they need moderate, extensive, or massive support. A plan is developed based on the initial rating and explicitly accommodates the need for care. Rehabilitation activities are offered as part of everyday life at the center, as well as twenty-four-hour care and support, in accordance with the Danish Service Law §85. As such, activities with social, physical, and cognitive characters are ensured by law. A daily training program is offered to maintain the acquired stabilization, and individuals frequently participate in various activities at the center.

The ecology of this setting is that its practices are enacted between care personnel, who are at work, and individuals with impairments, who are at home. This discrepancy of individuals coordinating actions at home and at work gives rise to interpretive considerations (Nielsen 2015, p. 272). The individual's permanent occupation of the site, versus the care personnel's occupation scheduled in intervals, has led to a principled policy that prioritizes and favors the individual's rights since they are living there; their habits and individual routines have priority. This decision is part of the ecology of the place. Other important aspects are the furniture, buildings, individuals living there, care personnel, family, peers, and research teams and clinicians frequenting the place.

Additionally, the center offers music therapy and is part of the Danish Network of Living Labs. A living lab is a cooperation between the workplace, in this case a residential care facility, and local education institutions. Research is carried out with the hope of improving QOL for the staff and residents, and with the aim of generating on-site knowledge within various fields about, for instance, practices evolving around living with ABI. Finally, this care facility is part of a European project, which enhances and engages local companies in the development of care technologies. In short, this site is a collaboration between a real estate owner, municipality, university, and several other project partners.

Third Circumference: Policies and Inclusion

In Denmark, inclusion is a main area of interest at institutions for persons with cognitive and physical impairments. Inclusion is understood as processual, which aims at securing adequate and equal opportunity to engage in social situations regardless of impairments. This ideological approach to inclusion is in accordance with the ICF model developed by the WHO. However, local practices of inclusion are subject to scrutiny.

Since rehabilitation has been decentralized, local governments outline a policy of inclusion practice in specialized care offers. The municipality's policy serves as pedagogical principle at the center. As a result, the board decides the required procedures to follow. However, several other procedures are predetermined by law. For instance, individual pedagogical plans must be created no later than three months after arrival to control the quality of the services offered at the center. This control is carried out in accordance with Service Law §141.

Generally, assessments of the standard of the services offered are carried out. However, out of the twenty-four individuals in the center, only one was interviewed during quality assessment. There are no details in the reports on the methods applied for interviewing individuals with aphasia and ABI. This is critical. Research into social inclusion of phase 4 patients is sparse. There are no national assessment criteria or guidelines for best practices of social inclusion of individuals with impairments; they are locally constituted. Although a national advisory board is in the process of developing such standards, for now the assurance of inclusion is the responsibility of the local board of the ABI center.

In an organizational perspective, a good deal of decision management is takes place without national guidelines. Inclusion is sought to be accomplished through local leadership, including the coordination of interests between the employed professionals and through the development of a local training program for professionals. The employees include many different groups of professionals: timetable managers, cooks, cleaning personnel, health professionals, and care teams. Additionally, other groups frequently enter the center: professional peers, relatives of individuals, press, and stakeholders.

As mentioned, several researchers, research projects, and areas of study are connected to the center through the Living Lab. Over time, many students, especially in medialogy,[6] communication, and musical therapy, have studied routines and practices at the center. Overall, the professional, pedagogical, technological, aesthetic, and physiological aspects of ABI have been observed and scrutinized in many respects and contribute to dialogues on practiced inclusion.

ZOOMING IN

Slicing Our Case Participant's Life

An EMCA-inspired interaction analysis demonstrated a slice of the social practices (Nicolini 2012, p. 218) that our case participant lived in his environment. In order to capture his perspective in an interaction analysis and formulate a person-centered praxeology, the personal perspective in interaction had to be accounted for. The course of the situated analysis is as follows. According to interaction analysts, trouble and repair in interaction reveal unspoken rules as they permit inquiry into other points of view (Jordan and Henderson 1995, p. 69). Therefore, this study sought to uncover the lifeworld of our case participant by orienting to corrective practices and repair in interaction. Two critical issues of correction between our resident and the therapists in interaction were analyzed. These issues are examined in a fine-tuned description, interactional consequences are scrutinized, and the findings and comparative findings are discussed.

Investigating Troubles in Interaction

As introduced in Chapter 3, the phenomenon of repair has been richly studied in aphasia. Repair is a broad term, generally concerned with the nature of turn-taking in interaction targeting the social organization of language disorders. Repair is regarded as a dynamic concept which brings the conversation forward (Schegloff et al. 1977). However, few studies exist on the procedures of correction in aphasia that provide a fine-tuned description of the distinct feature of interaction between therapists and individuals with aphasia (Klippi 2015), error-talk and error-fixing (Simmons-Mackie and Damico 2008, p. 5). The term "correction" is, thus, applied to target investigations of the psychosocial side of aphasia. Excessive correction in aphasia has proven to lead to emotional distress (Wilkinson et al. 1998). Repair is distinguished from correction by its analytical broadness as opposed to the concept of correction that refers to professional practice in speech therapy (Simmons-Mackie and Damico 2008). Correction relates to assessment of competence within speech and language pathology. For instance, the way in which words are retrieved, how they are enacted through gesturing, and how conversation is scaffolded (Clarke and Bloch 2013). This study, however, employs a different aspect of correction—the correction of knowledge, not correction of competence.

Two specific incidents of knowledge correction, distributed over two days of recording, have been chosen for this qualitative analysis. In the first incident, which is rich in organizational structure, our case participant claimed to have beer in his glass when it actually contained elderflower juice. A joint activity of inspecting our case participant's beverage resulted in a series of aggravated corrections by the therapists, resulting in the exclusion of our case participant from the dialogue. In the second incident, three complaints recur in three different interlinked sequences. In the second and third sequences, our case participant is complaining that the personnel at the ABI center are ignorant, similarly resulting in his exclusion from the dialogue. This incident is rich in resemiotizations. Interestingly, our case participant's complaint was located in a series of actions relevant to the ecology of this action. By ecology, this author draws on the integrational notion of contextualization, which is person-bound rather than sequentially bound, as discussed in Chapter 4. This sequence empirically demonstrates contextualization at work. Using EMCA and PT tools, our case participant's complaint was traced backwards from this local incident to a situation occurring one hour earlier when a therapist complained about the architects who built the ABI center. Then, the complaint is traced forward to the recording two weeks later, where, in a third sequence, our case participant was finally allowed to state his complaint. This is accomplished as a joint activity while reviewing the video from the first day of recording, which dealt with individuals complaining about the architecture of the center at several points.

Demonstrably, all three complaints were intertwined in our case participant's meaning-making. This is shown by our case participant's publicly available contextualizations of complaining in local interactions, in which the first incident was enacted bodily in orchestration with the therapist who was criticizing the architecture and the architects. Then, a new version of a criticism was verbalized by our case participant, but disregarded as a complaint in the second sequence. Finally, a third version of a criticism was brought forward in joint verbal and embodied orchestration between the research assistant and our case participant, resulting in his complaint being accepted in the third sequence.

The processual nature of these contextualizations are described in the analysis and characterized with the concept of resemiotization (Iedema 2003). As discussed in Chapter 2, this author understands and applies this concept experientially and individually, not structurally. Following an IL perspective, meaning is processual. Hence, it can never be encapsulated in language but resides in action, whether jointly or individually performed, and whether implicitly or explicitly perceived. As discussed in Chapter 4, in an IL perspective, meaning-making can be enacted momentarily, but meaning is never fixed because it does not exist as a linguistic construct due to the ontological IL principle of radical indeterminacy, discussed in Chapter 5.

Moreover, this study shows that correction of knowledge and correction of language are two different issues. The activities in the two issues of correction of knowledge treat our case participant not only as communicatively impaired; more importantly, and less fortunately, he is oriented to as cognitively impaired. However, this can be explained as a part of a professional corrective practice (Simmons-Mackie and Damico 2008; Wilkinson et al. 1998). Yet, this study's aim is not to assess the professionals but to investigate practices as they unfold in order to open a dialogue on the psychosocial consequences of practices of exclusion and inclusion in interaction in health and social care settings. In these incidents, exclusion is clearly accomplished by a joint series of aggravated corrections performed by the therapists' disengagement and their disaffiliation with our case participant's initial contribution. In sum, the practices in the two knowledge-correction incidents result in exclusion of an individual with impairment. Possibly, inclusion could have been afforded with an alternative perception of practice. An alternative perception of practice contributes to the employment of new communication strategies, and it ultimately supports changes of practice.

FINE-TUNED ANALYSIS OF EXCERPTS

First Incident: This Here Is a Beer

The following excerpt is an interaction between our case participant, Søren, and two therapists, and was overheard by a second resident and two researchers. It is valuable to note how his social role is constructed through the course of the interaction. ABI is not made noticeably relevant on the surface, yet the recurring social activities are bound to the implicit local construction of ABI. This becomes clear when we consider how our case participant is met during this initiated discussion. Therefore, the focal line is turn seven, where the therapists treat Søren as a non-ratified recipient.

We are on an excursion at a local shopping mall. We have just sat down at the tables to have lunch. Two residents and two assistants are sitting at one table while two researchers, who wear GoPro cameras on their chests, are sitting at another table next to them. A discussion about the content of Søren's glass arises. Just before this, one of the assistants, an occupational therapist, has been saying that it is Friday and that it is acceptable for Søren to have a beer. Meanwhile, the other assistant, a pedagogue, was away picking up the food ordered for Søren and herself at the counter (see Fig. 6.1).

After tasting it, Søren initially states, as we can see in the excerpt, that he has received a beer. The pedagogue responds with immediate orientation towards Søren in turn four, exclaiming, *"Er det en ØL?"* ("Is it a BEER?"). Her surprise is emphasized by her intonation in the pronunciation of ØL (BEER). The participant re-states a variation of his prior turn, *"-ja det"* ("-yes it"), maintaining that it is a beer.

The occupational therapist is increasingly turning the left side of her body and head towards the other therapist beside her, not looking at all at Søren. All the while, she is paying attention to the dialogue between Søren and the pedagogue. In line seven, the other therapist comments to the pedagogue, not to Søren, *"aj det er fordi jeg troede det var en øl"* ("no, it is because I thought it was a beer"). This could be regarded as other-initiated repair, as it repairs his statement with talk over his head by her saying, "*aj det er fordi* [...]" ("no, it is because [...]").

In turn eight, the pedagogue reaches out for the glass and smells the contents (see Fig. 6.2).

```
Participants:

S: Søren, our case participant
B: Bente, pedagogue
P: Pia, occupational therapist
PR: Pirkko, research leader
C: Charlotte, research assistant


GOPRO016 32:00-32:47

01  S:  ((points to large glass right in front of him))
02  S:  eh- eh- eh- eh=Ben[te det der det er [altså] en øl
        er- er- er- er=Ben[te this here that is a beer
03  B:                    [mm
04  B:  Er det en ØL
        Is it a BEER
05  S:  ja- det
        yes- it [noise]
06  P:  ((looks towards Bente))
07→P:  aj det er fordi jeg troede det var en øl
        no it is because I thought it was a beer
08  B:  [((reaches out for the glass. #Smells the content))
    P:  [((scratches herself by the mouth and looks over to Bente
          who is sitting with the glass))
    fig                                  #fig. 1
09  B:  Ne:j Søren
        No: Søren
10  B: ((nods))
11  B:  det lugter af hyldeblomst
        it smells like elderflower
12  S:  NÅ:hh nåh det- det- er-
        OH:hh well that- that- is-
13  B:  Det er så:n noget hyldeblomst
    B:  It's a sort of elderflower
14  S:  hm er
15  B:  æble=hyldeblomst
        apple=elderflower
16      noise
17  B:  ((takes the glass and looks down into it Smells again the
          surface of the glass from side to side))
18  S:  nå- så- der=kan=man=(se)
        well- there=you=(go)
19  B:  aj det dufter altså af hyldeblomst
        oh well but it does smell of elderflower
```

Fig. 6.1 Data excerpt. Søren states that he has got a beer, which cascades a series of inspections co-operated between the professionals and Søren

```
20  B:  ((takes the glass and reaches it over to Pia who is
        seated next to Bente))
21  B:  prøv og duft
        try and smell
22  B:  ((reaches out and holds the glass under Pia's nose))
23  P:  ((smells the glass))
24  P:  jo- jo
        well- well
25  P:  ((looks down))
26  P:  nej det er ikke øl
        no it is not beer
27  B:  ((puts the glass back at the table))
28  B:  Det dufter ikke af øl
        It doesn't smell of beer
29  P:  så ville der også have været bobler i
        then there would also have been bubbles in it
30  S:  Det- ja
        It- yes
31  P:  ellers er det verdens mest dovne øl
        otherwise it is the most flat beer in the world
32  PR: [HAHAHAHA
    C:  [HAHAHAHA
33  S:  det=dufter=da=af=øl
        but=it=does=smell=like=beer
34  S:  ((raises the glass and reaches it over towards Pia across
        the table))
35  S:  jamen det=bobler=også her
        but it=also=bubbles here
36  B:  [aj så ville der være så:n skum henne i kanten=hvis det var
        [well then there would have been kinda foam in the side=
         if it were
    S:  [Nå
        [Well
37  S:  ((COUGH))
38  S:  ja= ja
        yeah= yeah
```

Fig. 6.1 (continued)

In turn nine, she explicitly reveals his understanding as problematic (Schegloff 2001, p. 1947) by her statement, "*Nej Søren*" ("No Søren"). Her statement is initialized by a "no," demonstrating further affiliation with the occupational therapist by repetition of her previous turn. In turn eleven, she indexes that "*det lugter af hyldeblomst*" ("it smells like elderflower"). Then, she elaborates her inspection and, finally, a new category is produced in turn fifteen as a justification, "*æble=hyldeblomst*" (apple=elderflower). The inspection is supported with stepwise actions performed by the therapist. First, by taking the glass, second, by looking down into it, and third, by smelling the surface of the glass again, this time from side to side.

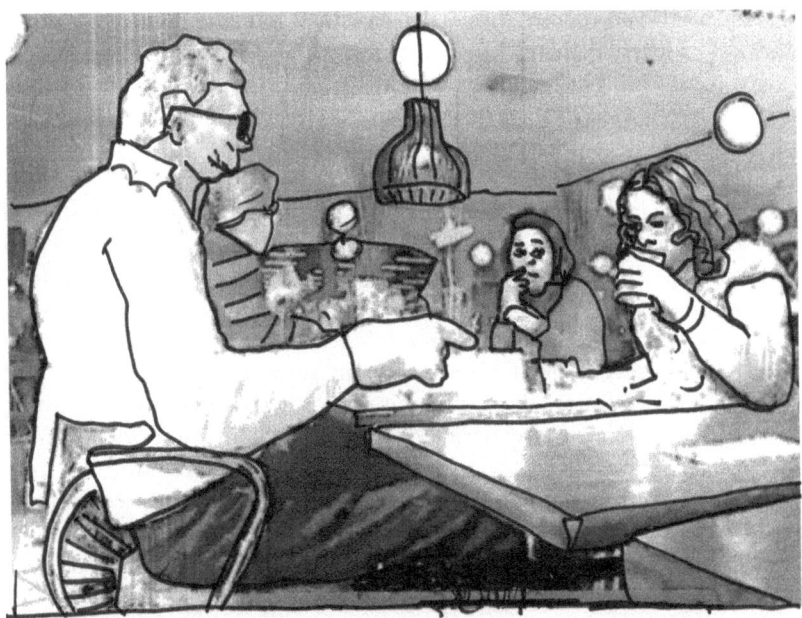

Fig. 6.2 The pedagogue inspects the glass by smelling it

Actually, Søren's response to this is compliance in line eighteen. The sequence could have ended here, yet, the therapist proceeds inspecting the beverage, so the response to his compliance is a continuation of inspections. Then, notice that the other therapist joins in and shows strong alignment as she offers a new justification in turn twenty-nine, "*så ville der også have været bobler*" ("then there would also have been bubbles in it"). Our case participant, again, halfway complies with a cut off, "*det–ja*" ("it–yes"), in turn thirty. The researchers affiliate with the therapist's designed joke in line thirty-one (that it is the world's flattest beer if it has no bubbles) with an adjacent laugh in overlap in turn thirty-two. Notice, then, that our case participant re-enters the dialogue and reverses to respond to the therapists with a counteraction, which he produces by stating, "*men=det=lugter=da=af=øl*" ("but=it=does=smell=like=beer"). Hereby, he aligns with the rules of the game, where accounts for perceptions of the fluid are made relevant. Thus, he intelligibly engages in the inspection gaming. In multimodality, food inspection and food assessment is considered formatted as other joint activities (Mondada 2009). The participant picks up this format and re-enters the dialogue by building on the recurring actions from the therapists (Goodwin 2018). This cooperative action is accounted for by the fact that the series is performed and formatted jointly between the two therapists and the participant.

Our case participant embodies his verbal contribution by raising the glass and reaching it (back) over towards the other therapist across the table so that she can see for herself as he adds a further justification, "*jamen=det=bobler=også=her*" ("but it=also=bubbles=here"). Notice that the therapist's *counter-response* leads him to give up the dialogue in turn thirty-seven. Finally, he resigns in turn thirty-eight with "yeah yeah." In consequence, the increasing determinacy of the beer results in his resignation from the expert indexers, leaving his intentioned motifs unexplored. Therefore, on the surface, the trouble source in this extract is the misascription of an object (the beer). This is accounted for with the beverage undergoing a variety of (extraordinary) assessments in this extract. Underneath the surface, however, something else seems to be at stake.

Experiential Correction

This part of the analysis investigates the participant's perspective more closely by extending the context in scrutiny of the focal turn seven. In turn two, the participant is pointing to the glass right in front of him as he, in that moment, makes his experience available. This sharing produces series of circulated knowledge gatherings around the lunch table. In line seven the other therapist employs an account for her attention, which is hard to interpret from this extract in isolation. Her comment to the pedagogue, "*aj det er fordi jeg troede det var en øl*" ("no, it is because I thought it was a beer") in line seven, needs linkage to a previous action. The occupational therapist was recorded talking about beer ten minutes prior to this incident. First, she commented to another resident present that it was Friday and, therefore, apt time for a beer. This talk was recorded while both Søren and the other therapist were absent. The pedagogue brought the glass to the table five minutes later, prior to the excerpt, and left to help our case participant. Then, Søren arrived in his wheelchair and was seated at the table. The pedagogue soon left the table again to pick up the food while the participant remained at the table. A dialogue was started by the occupational therapist. For the first time and in his presence, it was stated that this was a beer when the occupational therapist commented that it was great idea to have a beer on a Friday. Her statement was, however, repaired by Søren and by the research assistant who accounted that it in fact was not beer in the glass. This all occurred while the pedagogue was absent.

The response initiated by the other therapist in line seven, in this view, interprets as a resemiotization of her own understanding, which explains her discarding of the beer statement. Importantly, she verbally responds to the participant's initiative, "*aj det er fordi jeg troede det var en øl*" ("no, it is because I thought it was a beer") in line seven, but she solely looks towards and targets the pedagogue, not the participant, while accounting for her own previous mistaking of the contents of the glass. Crucially, she is talking over Søren's head. This tracing backward explains the way in which the beer is collaboratively constructed between the recipients in several reconfigurations. Yet, in the studied excerpt, Søren's statement that it is a beer is constructed as a trouble source, which needs correction and further meaning calibration. The series of corrections from line six and forward account for this joint interpretation between the therapists.

This excerpt demonstrates how the course of the unfolding interaction is driven by a typical series of corrections, which are made relevant by the therapists, and which the therapists now hold Søren accountable for. Notice that all Søren's inspections and assessments hereafter are disregarded by the therapists. The error of the beer is sought fixed during a long series of inspections of the beverage, correcting his misascription of beer to elderflower juice. This is done by positioning their inspections as objective (it is not a beer), and conversely by constructing his criteria as subjective (it is a beer). Though Søren, just before this excerpt, corrected the therapist's assessment of the beer, this action was never reassessed. Objective knowledge is orchestrated for fixing the participant's trouble-making. This is done by corrective inspections performed by the therapists.

As discussed by Trine Heinemann (2009, p. 2438), the exclusion of recipients affords the construction of them as third parties through not attending to them despite their co-presence. However, the therapists do not use third-person pronouns for our case participant in this example. Yet, the other therapist, through her visible bodily orientation and gaze directed towards the pedagogue, demonstrates that Søren is a non-ratified recipient. Notably, Søren has no one to support him in this sequence. This aligns with Parr's claim (2008, p. 20) that the significance of disabledness often produce an orientation from non-disabled towards individuals with impairment as socially incompetent. Interactionally, this is demonstrated by the therapists' counter-inspections in response to our case participant's participatory initiative between turns thirty-three and thirty-eight.

As competence, correctly produced knowledge pertains only to the therapists, resulting in a strong asymmetry which does not appear to be inclusive at all. In contrast, this example exposes professionals engaged in aggravated correction procedures, which afford the construction of our case participant as incompetent and cognitively impaired. Crucially, the outcome of the situation is our case participant's withdrawal from the conversation. Noticeably, he is oriented to as unaccountable. In consequence, he withdraws in turns thirty-seven and thirty-eight with a cough and a "yeah yeah."

SECOND INCIDENT: OUR CASE PARTICIPANT COMPLAINS ABOUT IGNORANCE

In the following part, it is anticipated that Søren's criticisms risk not being heard because they are disregarded interactionally. Demonstrably, our case participant's complaint builds on a previous action. His action is thus located in a series of actions relevant to his contextualization. Therefore, it is traced backwards to this initial action occurring one hour earlier, where the therapist was complaining about the architects who designed the kitchen where the first action takes place (see Fig. 6.3).

The following examples have been transcribed using a model inspired by Lorenza Mondada's multimodal transcription model (2014), since they are shorter than the previous example. The timing of gestures is relevant to this example, necessitating the transcription format being applied here. Gestures are transcribed in turns of talk, enabling an even more fine-tuned inspection.

Our case participant partook in this session where the occupational therapist criticizes the kitchen design as an architect's failure; hence, *the place* (metonymized) is stated for the first time in the recordings. We are in the kitchen next to the conference room. The therapist and the research assistant support Søren in tea preparation. Meanwhile, the

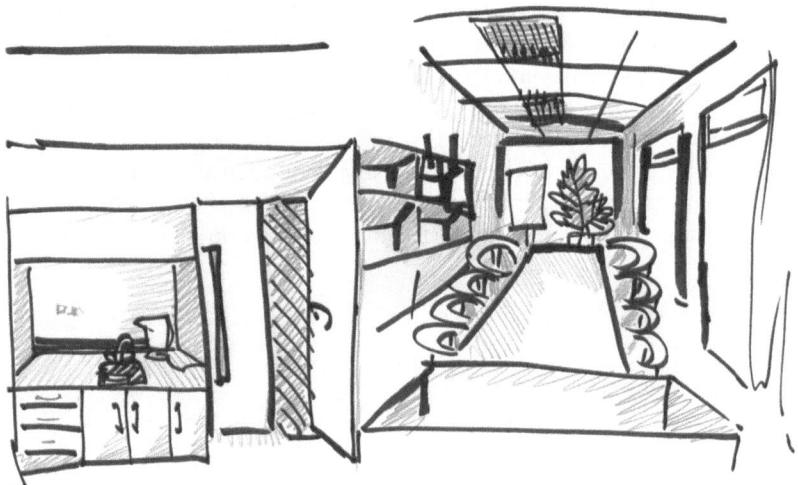

Fig. 6.3   The author's raw sketch of the scenes: The kitchen and the conference room next door

occupational therapist explains the pros and cons of the architecture regarding the kitchen design to the research assistant (see Fig. 6.4).

The initiative for the discussion is taken by the occupational therapist. She supports her verbal criticism by gesturing and pointing towards the surface of the tall kitchen table, demonstrating its hindrance to interaction for individuals with disabilities. Notice the cooperative orchestration of this action (see Fig. 6.5).

In line one, the therapist accounts for the relevance of the ergonomic problem of the kitchen design to the research assistant with a gesture while initiating critical talk, *"vi har lidt udfordringer med"* ("we have some challenges with"). At the same time, Søren embodies alignment with her. This is done by our case participant first facing his wheelchair towards her as she gesticulates, and then by rolling back and grasping the edge of the table that she just pointed to as he initiates enacting its insufficiency from line one until line thirteen. In line three, the therapist blames the kitchen design and, in lines six and seven, the therapist blames the architects for this design-failure, *"det er sådan lidt en arkitektfejl kunne man godt mene på et senhjerneskadecenter ikke"* ("it is sort of an architect's failure, one could suppose, since we are at a rehabilitation center, right"). Our case participant responds to this by reaching for the kettle, turning his body towards the occupational therapist (see Fig. 6.6). The research assistant verbally affiliates with the blaming in line eight, *"ja ja det må man da nok sige"* ("yes, yes, this is obvious"). The discussion between the therapist and the research assistant unfolds a coordinated talk of criticism of the architects who decided the kitchen design, which our case participant simultaneously enacts while attempting to preparing tea, for instance, supported by the lid dropping in line nine.

```
Participants:

R: our case participant
OT: the occupational therapist
RA: the research assistant


GoPro13 11.10-11.50

01   OT:    +vi har lidt *udfordringer# med
            we have some challenges      with
     ot:                  *gesticulates with hands, arms in sideways
            movement aligning table surface in the air--->
     fig                  #fig. 2
     r :    +approaches wheelchair, rolls back and grasps edge of kitchen table
02   RA:                          ja selvfølgelig
                                  yes of course
03   OT:    det er ikke alle (steder i) køkkenerne* der er  indrettet til det
            it is not everywhere in the kitchens that is   designed for it
                                           --->*
04   RA:                                          -ja
                                                  -yes
05   RA:    nej# det er de da ikke *særlig +godt -det
            No they aren't not very good          -it

     fig    #fig.3
     r :                        --->+
     ot:                        *turns to R and turns back to RA
06   OT:                                  -det er sådan lidt en
            +arkitektfejl
                                          -it is sort of an arquitect's
            failure
     r:                                        +reaches kettle
07          kunne man godt mene på et senhjerneskadecenter -ikke
            one could suppose since we are at a rehabilitation center -right
08   RA:    ja ja det må man da nok +*sige eh -ja
            yes this is obvious well -yes
     r:                                  +points at kettle while gazing at OT
     ot:                                 *approaches R
09   OT:    ja:+
            Ye:s

     r :      +touches kettle and takes kettle from dock and attempts at
            opening the lid
```

Fig. 6.4 Data excerpt. The therapist states the first criticism of "the place": An architects' failure

```
10    R:    ((noise)) (xxx)sikkerhed en vandkoger
                     (xxx)security a water boiler
11    OT:   -ja så er du på rette vej*+*
            -yes now you are going the right direction
      ot:                    *steps towards R with arms open to help and
            grasps kettle and holds it+
      r :                          +lid opens and drops onto the table*
      ot:                                                   *makes
            noise with porcelain in the sink
12    R :   -ja+
            -yes
      r :        +mumbles
13    R :   hvor meget kan der være i en+ (the) kande
            how much does a (tea) kettle hold
      r :                         +opens water tab$
      :                                  $water fills the kettle
14    OT:   hvor meget står der på den
            how much does it say
15    R :   eh max. 1,7 -eh der kan vel være en liter
            uh max. 1,7 -uh possibly about a liter
16    OT:   ja det tror* jeg
            yes that is what I think
      ot:             *opens drawer
```

Fig. 6.4   (continued)

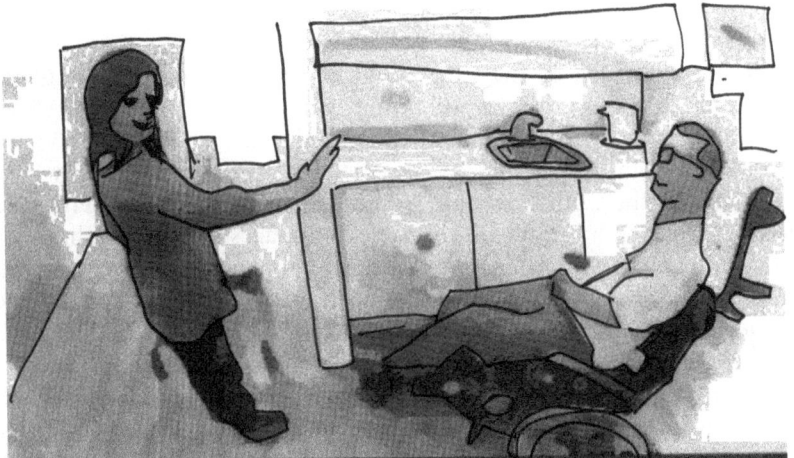

Fig. 6.5   Challenges with the kitchen's design are enacted by the therapist's hand gesture

In the excerpt, the therapist co-enacts with him, assisting him to reach and pick up items unreachable to him. He points towards the kettle in line nine as if enacting that the kettle is unreachable, indicating that

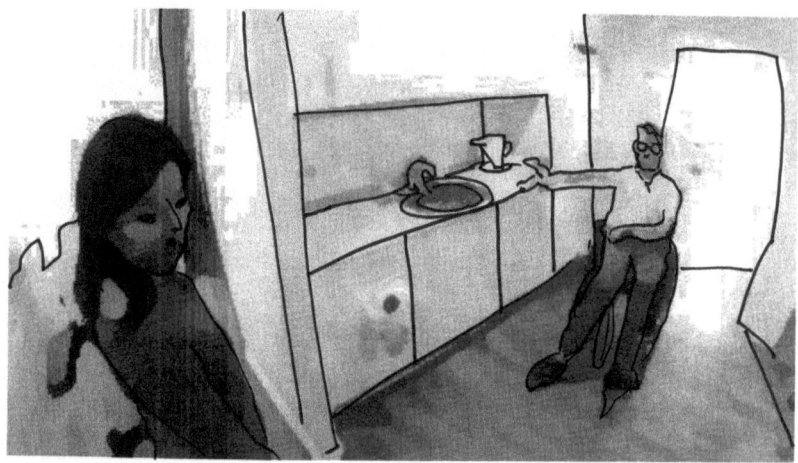

Fig. 6.6 The problematic architecture is coenacted by Søren and his grasping the table edge, and reaching out for the kettle

its position afforded by the table design is a trouble source. The therapist simultaneously orients towards him with a "*ja*" ("yes"). When he attempts at opening the lid, she scaffolds the action by verbally praising his effort in line eleven, "*ja så er du på rette vej*" ("yes, now you are going in the right direction"). She helps him grasp the kettle and holds it. Yet, the lid drops on the table and makes noise. Together they close this co-enacted, coordinated sequence of joint criticism. The tea prepared in this sequence is for the meeting that we are about to attend in the next excerpt. There, the place is taken up again as a building and then criticized by Søren. This excerpt centers on a ratified criticism with initiative taken by the therapist. Later, it serves as a semiotic resource, where our case participant states his complaint that he has been met with ignorance at the ABI center.

The Place Resemiotisized: I Have Been Met with Ignorance

This author now wishes to draw the reader's attention to our case participant resemiotisizing the physical surroundings from the example above in the following excerpt. The place is brought up as a point of departure for his criticism of its professionals. Prior to the excerpt, a round-table conversation about the ABI center and the professional capacities unfolded. Our case participant orients his contribution towards this talk. Notice how our case participant intelligibly builds on two things: First, the previous criticism of the place as he occasions it verbally, and second, the conversation about professional capacity. In sum, he reuses actions from past events as he performs a resemiotization of *the place as a building* as an entry for initiating his response to the professionals' praising. Hereby, he ends up discarding the professionals' praise with a subjective criticism. Again, the aim of this part of the interaction analysis is to focus the investigation on how our case participant is met when taking a critical initiative.

We are in the conference room, and it is the first day that we are recording at the center. In the conference room, the research team is introducing the project. We are several participants sitting at the table. Among the participants are residents, researchers, care personnel, and two occupational therapy students. In this excerpt, our case participant initiates his critical talk. Again, in this example, our case participant's shared experience is oriented to and constructed as insignificant, and he as authoritatively unaccountable. This becomes clear when we notice how our case participant is met in his shared experience by the therapist, who disregards him as complainant (see Fig. 6.7).

Our case participant spends a long time stating his case, stuttering due to his aphasic condition. Yet, over four turns, he states his experience of the place in one coherent stream of talk, only interrupted by tokens typical for individuals with aphasia (i.e., er, and), "*øh jeg studsede noget over da jeg flyttede hertil at at at man har lavet det her enorme sted øh øh og så og så øh og så har jeg mødt uvidende totalt uvidenhed om min situation*" ("er, I wondered when I moved here that that that this enormous place has been built er er and then and then er, and then I have met ignorant complete ignorance er about my situation"). He closely links the institution, "*det her enorme sted*" ("this enormous place"), in line eighteen with the fact that he has "*mødt uvidende total uvidenhed*" ("met ignorant complete ignorance") about his situation in line nineteen. By pointing at the therapist at the end of the table while producing the word "*uvidenhed*" ("ignorance") in turn nineteen, he links the building and its personnel. The meaning of the building is thus reconfigured and augmented from the surroundings to include the personification of the center (i.e., the therapist who is held accountable). This action is built in accordance with Goodwin's principled demonstration

Participants:

S: Søren, our case participant
R2: another resident
OT: the occupational therapist
cam: GoPro-camera attached to the research assistant's head

GoPro010013 03:29–04:16

```
17     S:     ø:h§ øh jeg studsede noget=over=da=jeg flyttede hertil at- at§ at=man
              e:h eh I wondered=when=I moved here that- that- that
       cam:   §focus on papers at table and refocuses on speaker
       cam:                                                              §turns
              towards other listening participants and returns to speaker
18            har lavet det her eno:rme sted=øh øh og=så=og=så-
              this eno:rmous place has been built=eh eh and=then=and=then-
       r2:    >>nods
19            øh og så har je-=mø:dt uvidende +totalt=uvidende
              eh and then I=have me:t ignorant complete=ignorance
       s:                                       +points towards OT
       ot:    >>looking towards S with right hand at her cheek
20            øh +o:m min situation ++ mm- øh
              eh a:bout my situation mm- eh
       s:           +points at OT     ++rests hands
       s:
21     :      (2.0)
22     S:     hvad kan det skyldes
              what might be the cause of this
23     OT:    hva- hva- jeg er i tvivl om
              wha- wha- I 'm uncertain
       ot:    >>looking down at the table hand at her cheek, raises head a bit
24            *hvad det er du mener (name)
              what it is you mean
       ot:    *moves hand in circles around her chin
25            *med uvidende
              by ignorance
       ot:    *hand at her chin
26     S:     men altså
              but well
27     OT:    men-
              but-
28     S:     men altså-
              but well-
29     OT:    men ellers skal vi tage* den senere **hvis det er
              but else we can discuss this later on if it is
       ot:                        *throws left hand with fingers spread in the
              air in circulation
       ot:                                      **hand back at her chin looking
              towards S
30     S:     eh ja+ lad os det
              well yes let's do that
       s:          +nods
31     OT:    ja altså den vil jeg gerne tage med dig senere ja ja
              yes well this I would like to discuss with you later on yes yes
32            det kan vi godt hvis det er okay
              we can do that if that is okay
33     S:     ja+ ja
              yes yes
       s:     +nods
34     :      (.)*
       ot:        *sinks, looks down, nods and winks to other participants around
              the table including R, hand around cheek
```

Fig. 6.7 Data excerpt. Second criticism of 'the place': Søren complains about ignorance

of cooperative action and the recurring reuse of past actions in human interaction (Goodwin 2018, p. 4). He combines elements from the professionals' praising of the center's capacity and the ratified co-enacted criticism analyzed above.

The situation is tense at this point. Notice how this is underlined by the movement of the GoPro camera, which is attached to the researcher's head. The camera movement in turn seventeen results in a significant pan back and forth in an attempt to pick up the other participants' reactions. After this, an interactional sequence unfolds over the next two turns with mutual repairs or incomplete initiatives between our case participant and the therapist (lines twenty-six through twenty-eight). All the while, the rest of the participants in the room are silently holding their breath. A significant pause of two seconds follows the completion of Søren's initiative (line twenty-one) which supports the tension of the atmosphere.

Since there is no response from the others present, Søren continues to elaborate his troubles and turns it into an answerable, targeting the occupational therapist he pointed at (line twenty-two), "*hvad kan det skyldes*" ("what might be the cause of this"). Now, notice how the delicacy of this action (Heinemann and Traverso 2009, p. 2381) is responded to by the complaint recipient, the therapist. Bodily, she orients to another resident in turn nineteen, seeking support and demonstrating that this trouble will result in disaffiliation. She then looks down at the table with her hand on her cheek and raises her head slightly (line twenty-three). Her orientation towards other recipients shows that she disengages with our case participant (Schegloff cited in Heinemann 2009, p. 2436). Finally, she verbally and multimodally targets our case participant's complaint straightforwardly. This next account blames our case participant for transgression, "*jeg ved ikke hvad du mener*" ("I don't know what you mean"). This is pronounced while she simultaneously is moving her hand around her chin in circles, demonstrating her disaffiliation with indexed uncertainty. By this response, she is verbally indicating that his answerable, indeed, is an unanswerable. In her choice of words, she reuses his phrasing. The significant part of her account addresses his lacking meaning-making, "I don't know what you mean," ends "*med uvidenhed*" ("with ignorance") (line twenty-five). This constructs him as non-ratified complainant as she demonstrates that she did, in fact, understand his complaint.

Our case participant with aphasia finds it hard to respond to this blaming of transgression. Notice how the inappropriateness of his initiative is responded to by her orienting to our case participant's sense-making, his knowledge of communication, as the real trouble source. Noticeably, she forces our case participant to enact his difficulties in communicating on a verbal level in the following, since our case participant is abandoned and unsupported with production difficulty for several turns as he is attempting at producing a new contribution to the discussion (turns twenty-six, twenty-eight, and thirty). By leaving him hanging, and by building on one of his attempts of reentering with a "*men*" ("but"), finally, the therapist takes over the turn and swiftly produces two chained turns, suggesting that they should discuss this more appropriately later on (line twenty-nine), "*men ellers skal vi tage den senere hvis det er*" ("but, else we can discuss this later on if it is"). Here, she verbally disregards the complaint by formulating a response which explicitly targets the inappropriateness of our case participant's complaint.

No one at the table engages in exploring what our case participant actually meant. This joint rejection from overhearers of his complaint is, therefore, supported by their silence. Rejecting a complaint is highly regulative. Even if the therapist's offer to discuss it later is a partial acceptance, she disaffiliates bodily and verbally with our case participant. In conclusion, she excludes our case participant in this excerpt with her course of responses to his complaint by applying two procedures. First, in the way that she disregards him, and, second, in how she purposefully leaves him hanging while he, obviously, is having production difficulties. The therapist's multimodal and verbal disengagement with our case participant's formulation is afforded by her recurring disaffiliation, by her long gaze down the table, and by her bodily orientation towards the other recipients clearly in the closing. This further shows the other co-participants that their engagement is irrelevant. She asserts our case participant's compliance to this even before he does, in the closing with two times of "*ja ja*" ("yes yes") (line thirty-one). He repeats this assertion with "*ja ja*" ("yes yes") twice more, mirroring her. This turn-taking is retrievable in CA literature (Schegloff and Sacks 1973). Yet, of interest in the analysis of this individual's perspective, this way of closing a discussion is found in several incidents between our case participant and the therapist, marking his resignation. She suggests a closing to which our case participant asserts with a "yes yes." In the above beer example, he withdraws with the variation "yeah yeah," which typically marks his withdrawal from the dialogue (Nielsen 2015, p. 268).

The Place Across Situations

The story of the metonymized place, however, does not end here. This section compares our case participant's resemiotizations of the place

```
Participants:

S: Søren, our case participant
RA: the research assistant
OT: The occupational therapist


GoPro020014 10:02-10:49

35    S:    hm+ @og- det kan man jo så undre sig over på sådan et sted
            hm and- it makes you wonder at a place like this
      s:        +gesticulates hand open
      RA:   >>arms crossed
      RA:        @raises arm and opens hand gazing at OT--->
36    RA:   og man ku jo ikke vide det hvis man ikke havde været med=ude og lave
            the@@
            and you couldn't have known this if you had not accompanied the tea-
            making
      RA:   --->@
      RA:        @@hand raised and index-finger at left chin
37    S:    nej nej øh+ hvorfor hvorfor har planlæggerne=arkitekterne så så
            no no eh why why have the planners=architects then then
      s:                    +raises hand gesticulating
38          ikke taget handicappede med på råd@
            not consulted the handicapped
      RA:                    @removes hand from cheek opens
            fingers in air pointing towards OT
39    RA:   mmm ja de::t er meget mærkeligt+
            mmm yeah tha::t is very strange
      s:                    +raises left hand and hits forehead
40    S:    =det synes jeg altså#
            I really think so
      fig                        #fig. 4
41    S:    det er hovedløst
            it is headless
```

Fig. 6.8 Data excerpt. Third criticism of 'the place': Søren and the research assistant discuss the problems they experienced with making tea with the other participants

and introduces his final contribution to this story. This next excerpt is included as it demonstrates our case participant's integrational proficiency in getting his message across. Looking iteratively across situations, our case participant applies creative strategies for conveying criticisms that he is building on the semiotic resources available in the situation, which are applied in his own public contextualizations. In the following, this is demonstrated by tracking the occasioning of the architecture and by analyzing its resemiotization (see Fig. 6.8).

Third Incident: Our Case Participant Criticizes Therapist and Architects

A third incident of criticism of the architecture arises. A new entry is made by bringing up the architecture in a response to a criticism on the recording being revisited, "*og det kan man jo så under sig over på sådan et sted*" ("and it makes you wonder at a place like this"), Søren

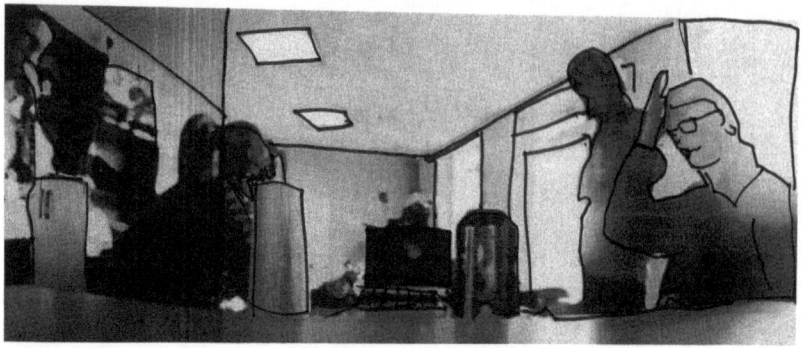

Fig. 6.9 Søren enacts the headlessness of the architects for not consulting the disabled by hitting himself in the forehead

comments. This initiative is immediately elaborated by the research assistant, "*og man ku jo ikke vide det hvis man ikke havde været med ude og lave the*" ("and you couldn't have known this if you had not accompanied the tea-making"). Notice that Søren simultaneously points at the therapist (line thirty-eight), as if she again represented the building, while he is blaming the architects verbally, "*øh hvorfor hvorfor har planlæggerne arkitekterne så så ikke taget handicapped med på råd*" ("why why have the planners architects then then not consulted the handicapped"). In this final excerpt, the place is resemiotized and elaborated by our case participant (see Fig. 6.9).

He hits himself on the forehead and states, "*det er hovedløst*" (it is headless). His contribution is not disregarded in this case.

In sum, the video recordings of the resemiotizations in the three incidents can be regarded interlinked because they have, one, been registered, two, been examined, and three, been demonstrated to serve distinct interactional purposes. The meaning of the architecture and the place is processually rendered in each excerpt. It is interlinked as it demonstrably is elaborated by the participants in collaboration. They seem to know what they are talking about.

First, the architecture is presented and discussed between the therapist and the research assistant with our case participant overhearing (turns one through nine). Meanwhile, this is indexed by Søren through his enactment of the troubles the architecture causes. This physically overlaps with their talk in turn eight, where he is pointing and calling the attention of the therapist. She approaches him, and together they demonstrate the inefficiency. Finally, the lid from the kettle drops.

Second, it later transforms into the episode where our case participant is first speaker in the excerpt in the conference room, criticizing professional ignorance. Notice that our case participant in the conference excerpt builds on the occasioning of the architecture of the place and makes it a relevant entry for his criticism. He states, "this enormous place has been *built*," but then he goes on to incorporate his own situation, building on a complaint, "and then I have met ignorant complete ignorance," possibly pointing to the professional ignorance he has experienced, *at* this place.

Interestingly, this story travelled on. Two weeks later, the team reviewed the data recorded with the two residents and an occupational therapist who were present during the first recording. A dialogue is initiated between a resident and the research assistant. The dialogue is inspired by the recording being watched by the participants. In the recording, the research assistant is telling a story about the tea kitchen incident from excerpt one, pointing to the fact that the kitchen is not designed for individuals with disabilities. Søren's intelligibility in complaining and criticizing the place when the camera is on is remarkable. This next semiotization of the place is made with strong affiliation from the research assistant. First, it is accomplished as a joint activity among the participants while reviewing the video from the first day of recording, which at several points deals with complaints about the architecture of the center. Second, it is accomplished multimodally with our case participant gazing directly into the camera.

Experiential Knowledge

It is remarkable that our case participant engages to the extent that is registered in the data. To him, it is a challenge to sustain a dialogue due to the condition of aphasia. However, the cost of not participating (i.e., silent compliance) is worse identity-wise (Nielsen 2015). Demonstrably, all three themes of the place are intertwined verbally. Furthermore, they show how our case participant communicates cooperatively and in a highly advanced way by orienting to the camera and informing this analysis, with or without the affiliation from his surroundings. He makes his lifeworld researchable by making his contextualizations in local interactions publicly available. In short, taking a praxeological person-centered analytical approach can make viewpoints available. These would be otherwise unnoticeable to strictly sequential EMCA analysts because of their limited perspective and their preference for studying sequences in isolation. Although there is some interest in ethnography (Arminen 2000), mainstream CA, emphasizing linguistics, prefers to analyze collections rather than longer sequences.

Including a Complementary Incident: The Newspaper is Wrong

The findings from a complementary incident of exclusion from this data set supports the above analyses and suggest ways to overcome unfortunate exclusion practices. Charlotte Nielsen (2015) discussed an exclusion incident with our case participant. Comparably, the co-construction of a past event with our case participant marked a critical situation, which led to resignation as a consequence of the therapist's disagreement with our case participant's experiential memory. This example is discussed in Nielsen (2015) and, like the above examples, demonstrates disagreement on knowledge entitlement. The topic in Nielsen's discussion is exploring what our case participant is actually trying to do. The disagreement centers around whether a journalist who covered a story of an event at the center had referred to data from the event correctly, according to our case participant's recollection. He states that the journalist refers to several points incorrectly.

Interestingly, the discussion about the article's data between our case participant and the therapist never explores his experiential memory. Rather, an act of persuasion led by the therapist treats the event as a matter of unnegotiable facts, like the above beer example. Facts are assessed by the therapist, who decides that our case participant's memory is insufficient, again questioning the accountability as in the beer example. Likewise, our case participant raises an issue and is targeted as the problem himself. The interactional result is resignation after the exertion of convincing the participant that his memory is deficit. Interestingly and analogous to the beer assessment, at no point does the therapist approach his actual memory to explore multiple descriptions of the event. Likewise, the activity of correcting our case participant's statements of his first-order perceptions of the beer in the glass or his criticisms of the place take up the whole attention of the therapist.

FINDINGS

At crucial points, social insignificance (Parr 2008, p. 20) guides the social orientation towards our case participant. He is held accountable for three things in the discussed data: First, the beer inspection series demonstrates him being excluded for subjectiveness; second, he is held accountable for not making sense when he is the one criticizing the place and, again, is excluded for his subjectiveness; and, finally, he is made authoritatively unaccountable for his own experience in a moment of an emergent memory of an event, which has been resemiotized in a journalist's story in the newspaper informed by third parties. Again, he is excluded for his subjectiveness. Following this, participation is made unavailable to him because of his subjective contributions, which this author suggests could have been met and tackled differently with a Wilkinsonian *let pass strategy* (Nielsen 2015; Wilkinson 2011).

This triangulation of IL and EMCA rethinks the analytical meaning of accountability since the IL concept of contextualization situates context with the individual stating what s/he considers relevant (Harris 2009b, p. 71). This is demonstrated by twofold tracking our case participant's attempts and failures at engaging in dialogues and by tracing his criticisms. In consequence, clear discrepancies between inclusion policies and practices were found. This called for a refocusing on the complexity of discourses and time-scales circulating sites of this local social action. However, this zooming out reassesses the first point in the interaction analysis. The norm is that therapists, family, and peers perform corrective practices with individuals who have aphasia, as in the examples presented above (Wilkinson 2011). However, consequences of such practices, at least in institutional settings, are not fulfilling the purpose of training, which is the strengthening of interactional participation.

The findings of this study are that, when supported by peers, integrational proficiency affords social and communicative stimulation. This was demonstrated in the third incident, the complaint about the architecture of the place, where our case participant is supported by the research assistant. Contrastingly, when participatory productiveness was not co-constituted and was hindered by the therapists, the consequences were crucial and resulted in discouragement, demonstrations of interactional and bodily exhaustion, and followed by resignation in the first two incidents (Nielsen 2015). These results were retrieved in this analysis.

Approaching Participation with Let Pass

CA analyst Ray Wilkinson specializes in interaction with individuals with aphasia. He recommends that therapists and peers support these individuals by setting interactional goals in order to change practices and enhance participation (Wilkinson 2011, p. 37). Corrections are (by these standards) highly problematic. Following Wilkinson, he suggests the exact opposite as an example of best practice. He suggests that therapists and peers do not correct memory and facts (Wilkinson 2011, p. 39). Instead, Wilkinson proposes to apply a let pass strategy (Wilkinson 2011, p. 44). Applying interactional tools in therapy and peer communication with individuals who have aphasia invites possibilities of inclusion practices. In conflicts such as the examples above, Nielsen (2015) points to the possibility of approaching our case participant's experiential memory differently on behalf of the therapist. Instead of correcting our case participant and treating his contributions as displays of deficiencies and impairments, the therapists could have chosen a let pass strategy (Wilkinson 2011, p. 44).

Treating our case participant's contributions as *relevant*, rather than *wrong*, would possibly have changed the interactional order. The demonstrated recurring corrective practices could have been replaced with a focus on other-directedness. For instance, by repeating his wording and by asking questions, the therapists could have encouraged him to continue his contributions. Furthermore, the therapists could have been more engaged with him, rather than with themselves and their own understanding. This would have created a solid basis for obtaining other-directedness, and it would have addressed the relevance of the important fact that our case participant shared his experiences. Nielsen (2015, p. 271) discusses a series of possible approaches that the therapist could have operated. What Nielsen does not realize and account for is the relevance of the actual encounter. The practices are corrective and the corrections happen for a reason. Nielsen leaves this reason uncovered (2015), as does Wilkinson (2011), who Nielsen leans upon in analysis.

The Crucial Consequences of Not Participating

The psychosocial consequences are not the only crucial outcomes. What may be conceptualized as *biosocial* consequences, meaning the physiological consequences of social activity, are important as well. The discussion of repair is central to CA and other interaction analysts. However, an integrational approach starts out by considering a different perspective in the sequence. As demonstrated above, it is not aphasia nor communicative impairment that is the central case in the excerpt.

In the first excerpt, the disagreement evolves around the assessment of a present object, the substance in the glass, which is circulated no less than twice around the table among its participants in a short but intense sequence. Søren may have initiated this disagreement for phatic purposes or for gaining an authentic response. And he might have very good reasons for doing so. After trauma, such as the brain injury our case participant experienced, habitually acquired knowledge about the world and self is impaired. Considering that Søren depends on the therapists because he has impairment and is living at a permanent care facility, the course of actions unfolding from participation to resignation are a devastating development which will mark his well-being both psychosocially and biologically.

Turning to Peter Naur's hypothesis in *The Neural Embodiment of Mental Life by the Synapse-State Theory* (2008, pp. 136–156), his review of William James' descriptions uncovers a mutual link between the physical brain and an individual's personality, which is managed through the development and rehabilitation of habit formation. This link is unexplored and overlooked within rehabilitation research. Habit formation requires constant cognitive and physical challenges in order to activate synaptic brain activity with the purpose of encouraging the brain to benefit from its plasticity features (James 1950, pp. 104–127). So, resignation, in this view, is for the worst, since participation encourages plastic benefits and develops the brain at the synaptic level.

We must not overlook that our case participant has a historical body of past and future communication routines with the therapeutic participants to draw on. In this light, disagreement could be a conscious strategy on his behalf. This might be his only way to provoke a real response in an extremely ordered and routine everyday life where he lives. Noticeably, several incidents like these are found in the data corpus. In the following section, correction is investigated and aligned with the beer example.

Making Corrections Relevant

EMCA can elaborate and approach the fact that actions happen for specific reasons. The analyst can start by asking what it is that actually makes it relevant to the therapists to initiate corrections of our case participant's contributions in the specific situation. In the first example, our case participant thinks that he has a beer, *perhaps* by mistake. He initiates the discussion of the beer. In the last example, he states that the journalist reported an event at the center wrong. Both examples lead the therapists to initiate a series of explicit corrections of our case participant's perception with the interactional result of explicit other-repair. Both examples end with our case participant's interactional withdrawal from the situation and interactional resignation.

In sum, the beer example and the example where our case participant's memory of an event is corrected share several interactional similarities:

- First similarity: Our case participant takes an interactional initiative.
- Second similarity: Our case participant is corrected and explicitly treated as cognitively impaired.
- Third similarity: Our case participant withdraws from the dialogue, resulting in interactional resignation.

The therapists perform some kind of corrective behavior in these situations. In sum, letting pass (Wilkinson 2011, p. 44) does not seem to be an option to these therapists. The signs that our case participant displays are treated as incorrect, and hence irrelevant, sign-makings (i.e., "it is a beer," "it bubbles," "it has foam"). In the above examples, the therapists clearly state in the first excerpt, "it is not a beer," and, in the discussed example from Nielsen (2015), stating that a journalist actually did get a story down right, according to the therapist's "correct" perception (Nielsen 2015, p. 267).

Perspectives on Repair

The rehabilitation paradigm in empirical interaction studies includes burgeons of significant findings from CA studies on language disorders (Goodwin 2003; Wilkinson 2011; Saldert et al. 2015; Rae and Ramey 2015). For instance, within the paradigm of CA, ways of co-constructing turns, ways of providing correction of one's own talk, and participant talk in conversations have been thoroughly investigated. In the classic studies, two primary ways of providing correction have been conceptualized.

Traditionally, a distinction is made between initiated and carried-out repair (Kitzinger 2013, p. 230). In the first case, the initial speaker's competence is supported by the proposition to self-correct by another participant, meaning that one does not generally correct another but allows for correction to the performed by the initial speaker. The initial speaker is the person who made the problematic contribution in the first place. Therefore, this phenomenon has been traced and described as *other-initiated repair* (Schegloff et al. 1977, p. 364; Schegloff 1992, p. 1331). Previous studies conclude that there is a preference for self-correction in adult conversations (Schegloff 1992). Furthermore, other-initiated repair categorizes as a more difficult mode of correction.

In the second case, which is the reverse case, corrections are performed by the co-participants. Here, repair is considered an aggravated way of correcting. The aggravation of the activity of other-correction is that it presupposes a lack of confidence in the initial speaker. Moreover, suspicion of incompetence is displayed. In this case, the second speaker does not trust the initial speaker's competence to perform a preferred self-correction. There are two main ways this can be signaled (Goodwin 1983, p. 658): it can be stated either as a manifest signal of the need of correction, or it can be done by the second speaker.

The consequence of the two ways of repair is crucial. Often, aggravated corrections lead to conflicts. Marjorie Goodwin's (1983) significant study on aggravated corrections in children's conversations describes language norms in conflicts. She describes the situationally appropriate norms governing language usage from adult conversations, drawing on Schegloff et al. (1977) as she singles out children's primary ways of commonly dealing with co-participants in conflicts. With this distinction between normative adult ways of correcting and children's *atypical* ways of correcting, she adds an interesting analytical perspective to the present data. Goodwin (1983) demonstrates that children's atypical conversation patterns are filled with variants of repair different from adult conversations.

As discussed extensively by Schegloff (1992; Schegloff et al. 1977), adult conversations have a preference for self-corrections. This is not the case in children's conversations. Conversely, children often perform what Goodwin labels *unmodulated* corrections, which categorize as aggravated repair. Goodwin analyzes how disagreement in children's conversations are accomplished by *counter-moves* (Goodwin 1983, p. 670; Jefferson

1987). Counter-moves are corrections which oppose previous moves. Perkins (2003) describes patterns in another type of atypical conversations. In aphasic conversations, repair is often distributed over several extensive turns. Children's conversations and adults with aphasia are not directly compatible since obviously these two populations have little in common biologically and socially. However, there are some common features in the organization of talk when the concept of speaker orientation is singled out.

Repair in the Present Data

The counter-moves that Goodwin (1983, p. 670) describes in children's disagreeing and the counter-moves that are found in this data set are strikingly common. The counter moves performed by our case participant in the first and the second incident, and the complementary example can be considered aggravated repair of the therapists' moves and vice versa. In a similar fashion that children accomplish disagreement in Goodwin's examples (1983), disagreement is accomplished here. This author's point is that self-correction does not have priority in any of the examples, whereas aggravated repair is present in all of the excerpts. The two seemingly uncommon groups share common interactional practices. Demonstrably, these organizational practices have consequences. Sometimes, the non-preference for self-correction has the consequence of placing the other in the membership category of incompetent. In this light, atypical interaction as a research program may accumulate strategies applied in diverse atypical populations.

Contrastingly, it may also be argued that no such thing as atypical populations exist, following the highly individual IL concept of integrational proficiency. Accordingly, the same interaction patterns are retrievable from distinct contexts with other groups of people. However, the wish to describe and evaluate the application of a concept such as *atypical strategies* makes sense. The question remains whether its falsification reveals the mythological character of the language concept applied.

AN INTEGRATIONAL ACCOUNT

To an integrationist, the presupposed, underlying understanding of language, communication, and sign-making constitute the very reason for the practices carried out. Therefore, part of the analysis is reserved for uncovering enacted language views. Interestingly, every sign created seems to stand for something specific in the therapist's practices. Grounded in our case participant's experience, whether or not the substance in the glass is beer is not something which can be discussed nor negotiated. To the therapist, either it is beer, or it is not. The representation of the sign in the form of a referential word (i.e., beer) can only be stated as a matter of right or wrong.

Our case participant's *experience of beer* (first incident, turn three) is not explored, but, rather, the referential sign-bearer (i.e., the object present) is assessed: a large glass with a liquid characterized as "apple=elderflower" by the therapist (turn fifteen). In the journalist example, it is not made relevant to uncover the significance of Søren's initiative, nor are inquiries into the workings of his memory made, nor into what makes him raise this doubt about the journalist's registrations of the event. Simply, therapy is initiated, Søren's memory is corrected, and the result is to stop him participating interactionally.

From an outside perspective, this strategy seems odd. However, there might be an obvious reason for the therapists to engage in the corrective practices we see unfold. If we have a closer look at what is being corrected, it is not a linguistic unit due to the condition of aphasia. Individuals with aphasia do not necessarily mind linguistic correction, but they do mind corrections of their knowledge about circumstances in situations (Nielsen 2015). This non-compliance to corrective practices of knowledge about circumstances in situations causes the repair sessions in the above cases, not other references. Further, the lack of effort to understand what our case participant meant by his criticism of the ignorance he claims to have experienced at this place proves an aggravated correction. In contrast, it is used to question his accountability and to construct a discrepancy between lived social inclusion which, unfortunately, results in social exclusion and interactionally framed unaccountability.

To the integrationist, creativity and proficiency have priority regardless of the infinite variety of modes in which they may be displayed. An excerpt from the data set discussed by Raudaskoski (2013) demonstrates how a female participant with severe ABI and aphasia is insisting over several turns and with explicit repair markers directed towards the therapist participant because the communication was of real importance to her. Apparently, the therapist helping her sign a consent document for participation in research was stating a wrong web-domain when co-constructing the speech from the female participant. This is corrected convincingly. As a result, the female participant manages to communicate her email address specific to the domain of Yahoo and not to Hotmail due to her insisting efforts (Raudaskoski 2013, p. 118). She proves extremely proficient in this example as she does not settle for less. She insists until determinacy relevant to her intention is accomplished. Unproblematically and because the situation is of real relevance to her, she intelligibly applies corrective proficiency with very few syllables but with strong interactional proficiency. Hence, her intention of making meaning is accomplished.

Yet, private contextualizations are not necessarily shared. The interjection tokens, *oh/yeah* (Heritage 1984), can mark that something new was understood but not spoken. Yet, accountability in social interaction is a spurious concept (Taylor and Cameron 1987; Harris 2009a)[7] since we do not share a common context in an IL person-centered view (Harris 2009a, p. 71). What, then, should we draw from our case participant's redundant closings, for instance. Noticeably, when he withdraws from each analyzed excerpt, his final contribution is "yes yes," or "yeah yeah." Certainly, he is not explicit about what this means; however, the excerpts convincingly demonstrate these are used interactionally. When this chained interjection occurs in each example, his participation is no longer sustained. The therapists do not make physical or cognitive impairment relevant verbally but interactionally. Basically, in a wider sequential perspective, his closings are repairing that he ever participated, as they state his withdrawal from a series of turns which accumulatively have constructed him as insignificant or present–absent, as hinted above.

As discussed by Nielsen (2015, p. 275), our case participant intelligibly applies a socially acceptable departure from dialogues. In this light, his resignations signify winning arguments through the action of resignation. This may seem counter-intuitive. However, this conclusion can be reached by applying extra-sequential knowledge. In this study, data is considered *objects of knowledge* (Ayass 2015) accumulated by collections and conducting longitudinal video ethnographic studies, which support the conclusions made. This is preferable to analyzing decontextualized extracts for inquiries into the general organization mechanisms of social action. Necessarily, a complementary analytical perspective is needed. A perspective less strict than the well-known sequential analysis from the traditional EMCA program needs to be introduced in order to study more closely what people are doing, viewed in a person-centered perspective.

A New Concept of Action

The application of categories in interaction analysis is currently scrutinized by alternatives to the CA concept of action (Enfield and Sidnell 2017). This author has pursued a different approach, which does not adopt the idea that language is at the center of social action (Enfield and Sidnell 2017, p. ix; Goodwin 2000). In contrast, this author considers communication to be the center of the analysis, based on the integrational proficiencies available and enacted in the situation. Indeed, language use is no guarantee for stabilizing determinacy (Harris 1998, pp. 81–83). In short, the communication strategies described in this analysis are not aligned with CA's analytical concepts, rather, these are applied for their visual properties for descriptive purposes. This is done by zooming in on the perspective of one individual in the interaction (i.e., our case participant).

This author is aware of several abductive elements of this analysis. Yet, as Scollon and Scollon (2007, p. 618) note, with a large corpus of data it is possible to investigate *the black box* of what is going on through observations of, for instance, similarly patterned consequences and individual interactional habits as demonstrated in this analysis. And, by abduction, assume the same mechanisms in function. When Charles Sanders Peirce discussed abduction as scientific method in his lecture *Pragmatism and abduction* at Harvard in 1903, he made a clear distinction between perception and abduction relevant to validation of the findings of this analysis. Abduction is, thus, applied concisely and purposefully in this analysis (Peirce 1995).

As stated in the zooming-in part of this analysis, the aim of this was to provide an alternative perception of practice. An alternative *perception*, thus, implied that the analyses of excerpts presented to the reader would afford a reaction. The excerpts and their analyses are now being aligned with the reader's experiential knowledge, which determines how the impressions from this author's analysis are perceived and reacted to by different readers. Logically, the perceptions cannot be denied; however, abduction implies that they can be denied because it is possible to question or even reject their validity (Peirce 1995, p. 169). So, when this author makes a triangulation between IL and EMCA in a PT framework, the reader may question the validity of this new joint approach. Notwithstanding this, abduction is incorporated in the pragmatic maxim (Peirce 1995, p. 176). Meaning, logically, that if this analysis is perceived as likely, then its hypothesis is automatically validated as an alternative perception of the practice presented. Possibly, this will afford a change of practice due to its perceptibility, its visibility, following Peirce.

The Validation of Difficult Partners: Integrational Linguistics and Ethnomethodology and Conversation Analysis

Multifaceted developments of participant perspectives within bordering fields exist.[8] According to IL, the EMCA participant perspective is describing the participants only on the surface, which does not include the lifeworld side of descriptive practice (Taylor and Cameron 1987, p. 114). Therefore, IL advocates would argue that person-centeredness in social studies is missing. Notwithstanding the divergences between EMCA and IL laid out in Chapters 2 through 5, the two approaches share many common traits and can work complementarily if some IL principles are compromised and data are allowed. At times, the approaches are even hard to distinguish from each other. Drawing on the discussion throughout this book, it is this author's belief that, together, the two approaches can support a person-centered participant perspective. However, a person-centered analysis had not yet been explored with IL, making this contribution relevant. As well, it is excused by its pioneering; this book is to be considered a conceptual work in progress rather than a manual.

This book has explored how two approaches to *meaning*, one being *private* and individualistic (IL), and the other being *public* and other-oriented (EMCA), can fruitfully be combined. To this author, the analytical contributions of IL and EMCA are intertwined. Foremost, theoretical and ontological disagreements mark their laminated divergence. To the integrationist, all communication is uniquely contextualized by the participants. This points to a distinct IL critique of CA's Achilles heel: The idea of presupposed normative accounts which generate analytical over-generalization (Taylor and Cameron 1987, p. 104; Enfield and Sidnell 2017, p. 9). The notion of atypical populations is a category (Antaki and Wilkinson 2013) that the integrationist, for instance, would argue does not appropriate the individuality of language impairment. A generalized category discussed by Orman (2017) is dyslexia. This disorder might cause trouble in sign-reading while it very well can be unnoticeable in conversation. Therefore, Orman argues that, to the integrationist, dyslexia as a language disorder does not categorize as a trouble in *the language* nor does it raise an issue of *fluency*, but it subscribes to a trouble with graphic-reading. By the same token, this author discussed in Chapter 3 that aphasia caused by ABI does not categorize as a communication disorder and it needs contextual reconsideration.

Yet, disagreements between IL and EMCA can be assuaged by further analytical debate. IL overfocuses theoretically on *language* and *the linguistic*, whereas EMCA, at least when applied in the study of language disorders, focuses on participation and action rather than language systems, which IL critics enhance (Taylor and Cameron 1987). This is clearly demonstrated by Goodwin (2003, 2013) who shows how a speaker with impairment, Chil, uses the ability of co-present peers to speak by co-constructing and indexing meaning cooperatively, accomplished through his varied prosody of a single interjection, "no" (Goodwin 2013, p. 11). Likewise, this is demonstrated in the example above discussed by Raudaskoski (2013). Refutably, these analyses demonstrate the structured organization of action conceived by the EMCA program. However, they also presuppose a theory of signs, since the accomplishment is an agreement between participants both with and without impairments and afforded by both parties' linguistic knowledge. Why else, then, distinguish typical from atypical? The problem for IL theorists is that they do not acknowledge the existence of any detachable linguistic faculty, which EMCA presupposes (Taylor and Cameron 1987). Rather, theoretically, they orient towards a program of individual experientialism (Pablé and Hutton 2015, p. 66). This explains why this author, carefully, applies the notion of resemiotization to visualize our case participant's explicit contextualizations of metonymized place, enhancing that the act of resemiotization is considered an individualistic enterprise in this analysis. In sum, divergences between IL and EMCA are not overcome but downscaled through the dialogue of this analytical probing.

Because of an inferior interest in linguistic and communicative norms, the impairment or non-impairment of the participants is of less relevance to the integrationist. Repeatedly, individual human proficiency is at the center of interest to the integrationist. Therefore, the IL concept of proficiency is in no way normative. It is highly individual and creative

(Harris 2009b, pp. 80–81), and it is motored by experiential indeterminacy. As discussed in Chapter 4, first-order experiences are driven by linguistic suspense of indeterminacy (Pablé and Hutton 2015, pp. 28–29, 59; Orman 2017). Surprisingly, this is demonstrated empirically by the fact that the entire room holds its breath when our case participant initiates his critical talk about ignorance at this place. Who knows how it will unfold?

CONCLUSION

This person-centered praxeology focusing on our case participant's habits in interaction portrays his integrational proficiency. Furthermore, this new analytical approach gives us access to a fine-tuned description of how individuals with impairment scaffold their social interaction by intelligibly drawing on basic interactional means rather than talk, extensive movement, facial expression, and haptics. In this view, this analytical perspective is a partnership between IL and EMCA, afforded by PT and video ethnography.

As seen in our idiographic analysis, the excerpts presented do not demonstrate communication trouble due to aphasia but interactional trouble, such as arguments, which can be ascribed to critical content of the communication. On this ground, the distinct contribution of this IL-inspired analysis is to give attention to and demonstrate how integrational proficiency is accomplished. For this, however, the integrationist will need to draw on EMCA in order to visualize descriptions and to avoid anecdotes and speculations as primary data. Therefore, this author largely appreciates observation studies that engage with individuals with impairment who have trouble making themselves understood by peers (Wilkinson 2011; Goodwin 2003, 2013). Hopefully, this analysis equally contributes to the psychosocial understanding of language impairment, however, by enhancing integrational proficiency.

NOTES

1. Here, materiality is widely understood, also covering embodied interaction.
2. This author takes responsibility for segregating while analyzing due to an urge to develop an applied integrational perspective, and seeking validity for Roy Harris's ideas outside the IL community.

3. See Chapter 5 for further discussion of emergent action and the notion of indeterminacy in an IL and PT alignment.
4. Goodwin's use of lamination (2013, p. 12). It is far-reaching and can be perceived to cover both here-and-now, moment-for-moment-building of shared action, but also the pasts that are present in situated action, semiotically and materially.
5. The research team share an interest in participatory activities. Overall, the common theoretical lens applied approaches the ability to participate in activities in everyday life in institutional settings.
6. Medialogy is education and research that combines technology and creativity for designing new processes and tools in media technology.
7. See Chapter 4 for an extensive discussion of this.
8. Apart from CA's participant perspective, for instance, Narrative medicine applies the narrative interview as a strategy to examine yet another participant perspective. See Chapter 4 for further discussion on participant perspectives.

REFERENCES

Antaki, C., & Wilkinson, R. (2013). Conversation analysis and the study of atypical populations. In J. Sidnell & T. Stivers (Eds.), *Handbook of conversation analysis* (pp. 533–550). Oxford: Blackwell.

Antaki, C., Billig, M., Edwards, D. & Potter, J. (2003). Discourse analysis means doing analysis: A critique of six analytic shortcomings. *Discours Analysis Online, 1*(1). http://www.shu.ac.uk/daol/previous/v1/n1/index.htm.

Arminen, I. (2000). On the context sensitivity of institutional interaction. *Discourse and Society, 11*(4), 435–458.

Ayass, R. (2015). Doing data: The status of transcripts in conversation analysis. *Discourse Studies, 17*(5), 505–528.

Cekaite, A. (2016). Touch as social control: Haptic organization of attention in adult–child interactions. *Journal of Pragmatics, 92*, 30–42.

Clarke, A. (2005). *Situational analysis: Grounded theory after the postmodern turn.* Thousand Oaks, CA: Sage.

Clarke, M., & Bloch, S. (2013). Augmentative and alternative communication AAC practices in everyday interaction. *Augmentative and Alternative Communication, 29*(1), 1–2.

Conrad, C. (2011). *Forståelseshandlingen. En empirisk afprøvet teori om narrativ forståelse som situeret betydning i dannelse.* PhD dissertation, Københavns Universitet, København.

Damm, B. (2016). *Sproglig betydningsdannelse i teori og praksis: En teoretisk og empirisk videreudvikling af det integrerede sprogsyn.* PhD dissertation, Københavns Universitet, København.

Duncker, D. (2005). Den integrerende kommunikationsmodel. In P. Widell & M. Kunøe (Eds.), *10. møde om udforskningen af dansk sprog* (pp. 137–146). Aarhus: Fællestrykkeriet for Sundhedsvidenskab og Humaniora Aarhus Universitet.

Duncker, D. (2011). On the empirical challenge to integrational studies in language. *Language Sciences, 33*(4), 533–543.

Enfield, N., & Sidnell, J. (2017). *The concept of action.* Cambridge: Cambridge University Press.

Glintborg, C. (2015). Disabled and not normal. *Narrative Inquiry, 25*(1), 1–22.

Goodwin, M. (1983). Aggravated correction and disagreement in childrens's conversations. *Journal of Pragmatics, 7,* 657–677.

Goodwin, C. (2000). Action and embodiment within human interaction. *Journal of Pragmatics, 32,* 1489–1522.

Goodwin, C. (2003). Conversational frameworks for the accomplishment of meaning. In C. Goodwin (Ed.), *Conversation and brain damage* (pp. 90–116). Oxford: Oxford University Press.

Goodwin, C. (2013). The co-operative, transformative organization of human action and knowledge. *Journal of Pragmatics, 46*(1), 8–23.

Goodwin, M. (2017). Haptic sociality: The embodied interactive construction of intimacy through touch. In C. Meyer, J. Streeck, & S. Jordan (Eds.), *Intercorporeality: Emerging socialities in interaction* (pp. 73–102). Oxford: Oxford University Press.

Goodwin, C. (2018). *Co-operative action.* Cambridge: Cambridge University Press.

Goodwin, M., Cekaite, A., & Goodwin, C. (2012). Emotion as stance. In A. Peräkylä & M. Sorjonen (Eds.), *Emotion in interaction* (pp. 16–41). Oxford: Oxford University Press.

Harris, R. (1998). *Introduction to integrational linguistics.* Oxford: Pergamon.

Harris, R. (2009a). *Integrationist notes and papers 2006–2008.* Gamlingay: A Bright Pen.

Harris, R. (2009b). *After epistemology.* Gamlingay: A Bright Pen.

Heinemann, T. (2009). Participation and exclusion in third party complaints. *Journal of Pragmatics, 41*(12), 2435–2451.

Heinemann, T., & Traverso, V. (2009). Complaining in interaction. *Journal of Pragmatics, 41*(12), 2381–2384.

Heritage, J. (1984). *Garfinkel and ethnomethodology.* Oxford: Basil Blackwell.

Iedema, R. (2003). Multimodality, resemiotization: Extending the analysis of discourse as multi-semiotic practice. *Visual Communication, 2*(1), 29–57.

James, W. (1950). *The principles of psychology* (Vol. 1). Cambridge, MA: Harvard University Press (Origin. 1890).

Jefferson, G. (1987). On exposed and embedded correction in conversation. In G. Button & J. Lee (Eds.), *Talk and social organization* (pp. 86–100). Clevedon: Multilingual Matters (Origin. 1978).

Jordan, B., & Henderson, A. (1995). Interaction analysis: Foundations and practice. *Journal of the Learning Sciences, 4*(1), 39–103.

Kitzinger, C. (2013). Repair. In J. Sidnell & T. Stivers (Eds.), *Handbook of conversation analysis* (pp. 229–256). Oxford: Blackwell.

Klippi, A. (2015). Pointing as an embodied practice in aphasic interaction. *Aphasiology, 29*(3), 337–354.

Laurier, E. (2014a). Noticing: Talk, gestures, movement and objects in video analysis. In Lee, R., et al. (Eds.), *The SAGE handbook of human geography*. London: Sage.

Laurier, E. (2014b). The graphic transcript: Poaching comic book grammar for inscribing the visual, spatial and temporal aspects of action. *Geography Compass, 8*(4), 235–248.

Legg, C., & Penn, P. (2013). Uncertainty, vulnerability, and isolation: Factors framing quality of life with aphasia in a South African township. In N. Warren & L. Manderson (Eds.), *Reframing disability and quality of life: A global perspective* (pp. 17–37). Dordrecht: Springer.

McIlvenny, P. (1995). Seeing conversations: Analyzing sign language talk. In P. ten Have & G. Psathas (Eds.), *Situated order: Studies in the social organisation of talk and embodied activities* (pp. 129–150). Washington, DC: University Press of America.

Mehan, H. (1993). Beneath the skin and between the ears: A case study in the politics of representation. In S. Chaiklin & J. Lave (Eds.), *Understanding practice: Perspectives on activity and context* (pp. 241–268). Cambridge: Cambridge University Press.

Middleton, D., & Brown, S. (2005). *The social psychology of experience: Studies in remembering and forgetting.* Thousand Oaks, CA: Sage.

Mondada, L. (2009). The methodological organization of talking and eating: Assessments in dinner conversations. *Food Quality and Preference, 20*(8), 558–571.

Mondada, L. (2014). Conventions for multimodal transcription (3.0.1. ed.). Retrieved December 5, 2017, from https://mainly.sciencesconf.org/conference/mainly/pages/Mondada2013_conv_multimodality_copie.pdf. (Origin. 2001).

Mondada, L. (2016). Challenges of multimodality: Language and the body in social interaction. *Journal of Sociolinguistics, 20*(3), 336–366.

Moss, P. & Dyck, I. (2003). *Women, body, illness: Space and identity in the everyday lives of women with chronic illness.* Lanham: Rowman & Littlefield.

Naur, P. (2008). *The neural embodiment of mental life by the synapse-state theory.* Gentofte: Naur.Com Publishing.

Nevile, M. (2015). The embodied turn in research on language and social interaction. *Research on Language and Social Interaction, 48*(2), 121–151.

Nicolini, D. (2009). Zooming in and out: Studying practices by switching theoretical lenses and trailing connections. *Organization Studies, 30*(12), 1391–1418.

Nicolini, D. (2012). *Practice theory, work, and organization—An introduction.* Oxford: Oxford University Press.

Nielsen, C. (2011). Towards applied integrationism: Integrating autism in teaching and coaching Sessions. *Language Sciences, 33*(4), 593–602.

Nielsen, C. (2015). Senhjerneskade i et forståelsesperspektiv. In S. Frimann, M. Sørensen, & H. Wentzer (Eds.), *Sammenhænge i sundhedskommunikation* (pp. 247–281). Aalborg: Aalborg Universitetsforlag.

Orman, J. (2017). Indeterminacy in sociolinguistics and integrationist theory. In A. Pablé (Ed.), *Critical humanist perspectives: The integrational turn in philosophy of language and communication* (pp. 96–113). London: Routledge.

Pablé, A., & Hutton, C. (2015). *Signs, meaning and experience.* Berlin: De Gruyter Mouton.

Parr, H. (2008). *Mental health and social space: Towards inclusionary geographies?* Oxford: Blackwell.

Peirce, C. (1995). Pragmatisme og abduktion. In L. Andersen (Trans.), *Semiotik og pragmatisme* (pp. 163–178). København: Gyldendal (Origin. 1903).

Perkins, L. (2003). Negotiating repair in aphasic conversation: Interactional issues. In C. Goodwin (Ed.), *Conversation and brain damage* (pp. 147–162). Oxford: Oxford University Press.

Rae, J., & Ramey, M. (2015). Parents resources for facilitating the activities of children with autism at home. In J. N. Lester & M. O'Reilly (Eds.), *The Palgrave handbook of child mental health: Discourse and conversation studies* (pp. 459–479). Basingstoke: Palgrave Macmillan.

Raudaskoski, P. (1999). *The use of communicative resources in language technology environments: A conversation analytic approach to semiosis at computer media.* PhD dissertation, University of Oulu, Oulu.

Raudaskoski, P. (2013). From understanding to participation: A relational approach to embodied practices. In T. Keisanen, E. Kärkkäinen, M. Rauniomaa, P. Siitonen, & M. Siromaa (Eds.), *Multimodal discourses of participation, AfinLA yearbook* (Vol. 71, pp. 103–121). Jyväskylä: Suomen Soveltavan Kielitieteen Yhdistyks (AFinLA).

Sacks, H., Schegloff, E., & Jefferson, G. (1974). A simplest systematics for the organization of turn-taking for conversation. *Language, 50*(4), 696–735.

Saldert, C., Johansson, C., & Wilkinson, R. (2015). An interaction-focused intervention approach to training everyday communication partners: A single case study. *Aphasiology, 29*(3), 378–399.

Sarangi, S. (2007). The anatomy of interpretation: Coming to terms with the analyst's paradox in professional discourse studies. *Text and Talk, 27*(5/6), 567–584.

Schatzki, T. (2013). Activity as an indeterminate social event. In S. Reynolds, D. Egan, & A. Weneland (Eds.), *Wittgenstein and Heidegger: Pathways and provocations* (pp. 179–194). London: Routledge.

Schegloff, E. (1992). Repair after next turn: The last structurally provided defense of intersubjectivity in conversation. *American Journal of Sociology, 97*(5), 1295–1345.

Schegloff, E. (2001). Getting serious: Joke -> serious 'no' ✩. Squib. *Journal of Pragmatics, 33,* 1947–1955. https://doi.org/10.1016/S0378-2166(00)00073-4.

Schegloff, E., & Sacks, H. (1973). Opening up closings. *Semiotica, 8*(4), 289–327.

Schegloff, E., Sacks, H., & Jefferson, G. (1977). The preference for self-correction in the organization of repair in conversation. *Language, 53*(2), 361–382.

Scollon, R., & Scollon, S. W. (2004). *Discourse and the emerging internet.* London: Routledge.

Scollon, R., & Scollon, S. W. (2007). Nexus analysis: Refocusing ethnography on action. *Journal of Sociolinguistics, 11*(5), 608–625.

Simmons-Mackie, N., & Damico, J. (2008). Exposed and embedded corrections in aphasia therapy: Issues of voice and identity. *International Journal of Language and Communication Disorders, 43*(1), 5–17.

Taylor, T., & Cameron, D. (1987). *Analysing conversation—Rules and units in the structure of talk.* Oxford: Pergamon Press.

ten Have, P. (2004). *Understanding qualitative research and ethnomethodology.* London: Sage.

Wallace, S., Worrall, L., Rose, T., Dorze, G., Isaksen, J., Pak, A., et al. (2016). Which outcomes are most important to people with aphasia and their families? An international nominal group technique study framed within the ICF. *Disability and Rehabilitation, 39*(14), 1–16.

Wilkinson, R. (2011). Changing interactional behavior: Using conversation analysis in intervention programmes for aphasic conversation. In C. Antaki (Ed.), *Applied conversation analysis: Intervention and change in institutional talk* (pp. 32–53). Basingstoke: Palgrave Macmillan.

Wilkinson, R., Bryan, K., Lock, S., Bayley, K., Maxim, J., Bruce, C., et al. (1998). Therapy using conversation analysis: Helping couples adapt to aphasia in conversation. *International Journal of Language and Communication Disorders, 33,* 144–149.

Worsøe, L. (2014). *Nye ord på nye måder: Nyorddannelse belyst fra et dynamisk sprog- og kognitionssyn.* PhD dissertation, Københavns Universitet, København.

CHAPTER 7

Conclusion

Abstract Modern health and social care defines itself as patient-centered and other-oriented, at least ideologically (Sarangi in Text and Talk 27:567–584, 2007). This book's analytical approach aligns with this discursive turn. In consequence, the experiential side of health and social care has been sought explored. Social practice studies have contributed to conceptualizing a participant perspective analytically (Sacks et al. in Language 50:696–735, 1974; Schegloff in Am. J. Sociol. 97:1295–1345, 1992). However, this book has conceptualized a participant perspective based on an IL–PT-inspired ontology, which distinctly contextualizes the individual participant perspective.

Keywords Patient-centeredness · Other-orientation
Health and social care New participants' perspective · Integrational
linguistics

In this book, aphasia and acquired brain injury (ABI) have been approached as a person's qualitatively different life-world. This approach agrees with current trends in language disorders of informing the development of quality of life (QOL) for individuals with impairments (Isaksen and Brouwe 2015; Wallace et al. 2016), and suggest following the International Classification of Functioning, Disability And Health (ICF) model developed by the WHO. As discussed in Chapter 3, traditionally, studies in language disorders followed a clinical discourse. In neurological approaches (Baron-Cohen 1995; Frith 2003), the processor in persons with language disorders and ABI is considered broken. However, interaction studies with a detailed understanding of action have shown that individuals with impairments often do not behave according to their diagnosis. Studies decipher that several competences are overlooked (Dickerson et al. 2005; Goodwin 2003; Nielsen 2011; Sterponi 2004). In contrast to clinical approaches, this conceptualization of language impairment requires the analyst to phenomenologically align with the impaired individuals, since to understand is a *sign-making business* which is co-operated between participants, not decoded by broken processors (Goodwin 2013; Nielsen 2011; Wilkinson et al. 2011). Here, individuals with aphasia and ABI are assumed to know a great deal more than clinicians, psychologists, or therapists may assume. Therefore, research with the participants in their everyday settings is recommended and encouraged for development of QOL instead of testing the participants' competences in a decontextualized manner.

In a person-centered praxeology, the analyst should try to understand the participants' categories rather than presuppose categories in advance. This can be done by careful noticing and long-term engaged observation. The analyst must try to understand the expressions and actions being displayed from his or her knowledge and acquaintance with the participants, which he or she should take time to get to know and follow over a period of time. Rather than depending on a pre-established analytical system based on structural strategy rules and normativity, creativity and unique aspects of the participation abilities of individuals should be investigated to enhance development of new skills in social practice proficiency. This discourse of understanding the individual is needed to supplement a clinical discourse in rehabilitation of language and communication.

This study's empirical contribution is, thus, a pioneering attempt to describe and discuss a new theoretical and methodological framework of everyday interaction: the emergent nature of everyday organizational and social life, momentary meanings, bodies, minds, things, knowledge, discourses, structures, agency, identities, and other entities or processes that are accomplished and resemiotized by participants who cooperatively reconfigure meaning in the ongoing stream of social practices. The descriptive analysis uncovered how troubles in interaction were oriented to and accomplished. Communicative patterns of inclusion and exclusion were scrutinized in sample analyses from the data collection of video-recorded troubles in everyday interaction. Furthermore, suggestions were made for an alternative perception of the troubles.

The new analytical perspective probes a participants' perspective as a matter of agency linked to the activity of contextualizing rather than focusing on the traditional mechanisms and logistics of the interaction. This study's focus attends to the way in which orienting to trouble caused by expected memory problems is part of inclusion or exclusion practices. The analysis benefitted from the tools offered by ethnomethodology and conversation analysis program (EMCA). Yet, the ontologies of IL and PT have a more fine-tuned understanding of emergent practices.

REFERENCES

Baron-Cohen, S. (1995). *Mindblindness: An essay on autism and theory of mind.* Cambridge, MA: MIT Press.

Dickerson, P., Rae, J., Stribling, P., Dautenhahn, K., & Werry, I. (2005). Autistic children's co-ordination of gaze and talk: Re-examining the "asocial" autist. In K. Richards & P. Seedhouse (Eds.), *Applying conversation analysis* (pp. 19–37). Basingstoke: Palgrave Macmillan.

Frith, U. (2003). *Autism: Explaining the enigma* (2nd ed.). Oxford: Blackwell.

Goodwin, C. (Ed.). (2003). *Conversation and brain damage.* Oxford: Oxford University Press.

Goodwin, C. (2013). The co-operative, transformative organization of human action and knowledge. *Journal of Pragmatics, 46*(1), 8–23.

Isaksen, J., & Brouwer, C. (2015). Assessments in outcome evaluation in aphasia therapy: Substantiating the claim. *Journal of International Research in Communication Disorders, 6*(1), 71–95.

Nielsen, C. (2011). Towards applied integrationism: Integrating autism in teaching and coaching sessions. *Language Sciences, 33*(4), 593–602.

Sacks, H., Schegloff, E., & Jefferson, G. (1974). A simple systematics for the organization of turn-taking for conversation. *Language, 50*(4), 696–735.

Sarangi, S. (2007). The anatomy of interpretation: Coming to terms with the analyst's paradox in professional discourse studies. *Text and Talk, 27*(5/6), 567–584.

Schegloff, E. (1992). Repair after next turn: The last structurally provided defense of intersubjectivity in conversation. *American Journal of Sociology, 97*(5), 1295–1345.

Sterponi, L. (2004). Construction of rules, accountability and moral identity by high-functioning children with autism. *Discourse Studies, 6*, 207–228.

Wallace, S., Worrall, L., Rose, T., Dorze, G., Isaksen, J., Pak, A., et al. (2016). Which outcomes are most important to people with aphasia and their families? An international nominal group technique study framed within the ICF. *Disability and Rehabilitation, 39*(14), 1–16.

Wilkinson, R., Lock, S., Bryan, K., & Sage, K. (2011). Interaction-focused intervention for acquired language disorders: Facilitating mutual adaptation in couples where one partner has aphasia. *International Journal of Speech-Language Pathology, 13*(1), 74–87.

INDEX